MOLECULES THAT MATTER

An Integrative Approach to Biomolecular Science

By

ABDUS SALAM

DISCLAIMER

PRINTING HISTORY
First Edition — 2026

Table of Contents

Preface

This book was born from a conviction: that the molecular world the world of proteins, DNA, lipids, carbohydrates, and their countless interactions is not only scientifically important but genuinely thrilling. The molecules that build, power, protect, and govern every living thing are objects of extraordinary elegance, and the story of how we came to understand them is one of the greatest intellectual adventures in the history of science.

Molecules That Matter: An Integrative Approach to Biomolecular Science is designed to be both rigorous and readable a text that does not sacrifice depth for accessibility, nor engagement for precision. It is written for students of biochemistry, molecular biology, and the life sciences at the undergraduate and postgraduate level, as well as for scientifically minded general readers who wish to understand life at its molecular foundations.

The book is organized into twelve chapters, progressing from the chemical foundations of biology through the four major classes of biomolecules, then into the dynamic processes of metabolism and gene expression, and finally to the applications of biomolecular knowledge in medicine and the frontiers of current research. Each chapter is written as a self-contained narrative beginning with a scene-setting introduction, proceeding through detailed treatment of the chapter's core topics, and concluding with a summary that consolidates the key concepts.

A note on style: I have deliberately written this book in an engaged, narrative voice rather than the dry, declarative style of many textbooks. I believe that science is best communicated as the human story that it is a story of curiosity, creativity, surprise, and the sheer joy of understanding. The facts and concepts in these pages are fully scientifically rigorous; the prose in which they are presented aims to be as vivid as the science warrants.

I am grateful to the generations of scientists whose work is described in these pages, and to the students whose questions have sharpened my thinking. Any errors or omissions are, of course, entirely my own.

— Abdus Salam

INTRODUCTION

The Invisible Architecture of Life

Why biomolecules matter and why they should fascinate you

You are, at this moment, approximately 37 trillion cells, each one a sealed universe of staggering complexity. Inside every one of those cells, tens of thousands of distinct molecular machines are at work reading DNA, building proteins, generating energy, repairing damage, signaling to neighbors, defending against invaders, and maintaining the precise chemical conditions that separate life from non-life. You are not merely made of molecules. You are, in the most literal and meaningful sense, a community of molecules organized, communicating, and cooperating across scales of complexity that exceed anything human engineers have yet managed to design.

This book is about those molecules the four great families of biological macromolecules that constitute the molecular architecture of every living thing on Earth. Carbohydrates, lipids, proteins, and nucleic acids are not merely the subject matter of biochemistry textbooks. They are the substance of memory and movement, of growth and decay, of illness and healing. They are the molecules that carry the instructions for building every organism that has ever lived. They are the catalysts that make chemistry possible at the temperatures and conditions compatible with life. They are the membranes that define the boundary between self and world. They are the signals that allow cells to talk to one another across the vast social networks of the body.

To study biomolecules is not to reduce life to mere chemistry it is to discover that chemistry, at a sufficient level of organization, becomes life. And that discovery, made over two centuries of increasingly precise and powerful investigation, is one of the most profound and humbling insights that science has ever produced.

I.

Why Molecules? Why Now?

The history of biology is, in one sense, the history of scale. For thousands of years, biologists worked at the scale of the whole organism describing anatomy, cataloguing species, observing behavior. In the seventeenth century, the invention of the microscope opened the scale of the cell revealing a hidden world of microorganisms, cellular structure, and the fundamental unit of life. In the twentieth century, a new set of tools X-ray crystallography, electron microscopy, ultracentrifugation, chromatography, electrophoresis, and eventually DNA sequencing and cryo-EM opened the molecular scale. For the first time, biologists could see not just the cell but the individual molecules that made the cell work.

What they found at the molecular scale was not a simple, mechanical system. It was something far more extraordinary a dynamic, self-organizing, self-repairing, information-processing network of almost unimaginable intricacy. A single human cell contains approximately 42 million protein molecules, representing around 10,000 distinct protein types, interacting in networks of extraordinary complexity. The human genome contains roughly 3.2 billion base pairs of DNA, encoding approximately 20,000 protein-coding genes, plus tens of thousands of non-coding RNA genes whose functions are still being discovered. The metabolic network of the cell encompasses thousands of distinct chemical reactions, each catalyzed by a specific enzyme, precisely regulated in response to the cell's current needs.

And yet this is perhaps the most remarkable fact of all all of this complexity is built from a surprisingly small chemical toolkit. Twenty amino acids. Four nucleotide bases. A handful of monosaccharide units. A few dozen fatty acid types. From these limited chemical alphabets, the entire diversity of life from bacteria to blue whales, from viruses to redwood trees is constructed.

This economy of means is not an accident. It reflects the logic of evolution, which builds complex systems by combining simple, reliable components in an ever-increasing variety of arrangements. Understanding those components the molecules of life is the foundation of understanding all biology, all medicine, all biotechnology. This is why molecules matter. This is why, at this particular moment in scientific history when our ability to read, edit, and even write genomes is transforming everything from agriculture to medicine to our understanding of human identity the study of biomolecules has never been more important or more urgent.

II.

The Four Families: A Brief Overview

The four major classes of biomolecules carbohydrates, lipids, proteins, and nucleic acids are each introduced here in outline, as a preview of the detailed treatment in the chapters ahead. Think of this as a first meeting: an introduction, not an education. The education comes chapter by chapter, section by section, molecule by molecule, as we explore each family in depth.

Carbohydrates are the sugars and their polymers the molecular fuel of cellular metabolism, the structural scaffolding of plant cell walls, and the identity tags on the surfaces of cells. Glucose, the six-carbon sugar that powers almost all cellular energy generation, is perhaps the single most important small molecule in biology. Cellulose built from glucose linked in a different way is the most abundant organic molecule on Earth. The difference between these two molecules, which have identical chemical formulas, comes down to a single bond angle. This is the kind of detail that makes biochemistry both maddening and magnificent: tiny structural differences with enormous functional consequences.

Lipids are the hydrophobic molecules the oils, fats, waxes, and steroids that define the boundaries of cells through the lipid bilayer, store energy in dense, anhydrous form in adipose tissue, and carry some of the most potent molecular signals in the body. The lipid bilayer the self-assembling, fluid, selectively permeable membrane that surrounds every cell is one of the most elegant structures in all of biology: a structure that arises spontaneously from the chemistry of amphipathic molecules, requiring no template and no instruction, driven purely by thermodynamics.

Proteins are the molecular workhorses of the cell arguably the most versatile and important class of biomolecules. Enzymes are proteins. Antibodies are proteins. The motor proteins that drive muscle contraction are proteins. The channels through which ions cross cell membranes are proteins. The structural fibers of skin, hair, and connective tissue are proteins. The receptors that sense hormones, neurotransmitters, and light are proteins. The machines that replicate DNA, transcribe genes, and translate mRNA are complexes of proteins and RNA. If carbohydrates are the fuel and lipids are the membranes, proteins are the engines, the gatekeepers, the workers, and the architects of cellular life.

Nucleic acids DNA and RNA are the information molecules of life. DNA stores the genetic instructions for building every protein and regulating every cellular process. RNA carries those instructions from the nucleus to the cytoplasm, translates them into protein sequences, catalyzes critical reactions (as ribozymes), and regulates gene expression (as microRNAs, siRNAs, and long non-coding RNAs). The story of how we came to understand nucleic acids from Miescher's isolation of nuclein in 1869, through

Griffith's transformation experiments, Avery's identification of DNA as the transforming principle, the Watson-Crick double helix, the cracking of the genetic code, and the CRISPR revolution is one of the most dramatic and consequential narratives in the history of science.

III.

The Architecture of This Book

This book is organized into twelve chapters, each devoted to a major topic in biomolecular science. The chapters are arranged to build understanding progressively foundational chemistry first, then the major biomolecule classes, then the dynamic processes that use them, then the applications of biomolecular knowledge in medicine and the frontiers of current research.

Chapter 1 establishes the chemical foundations: the six key elements of biology, the remarkable properties of water, the functional groups that give biomolecules their chemical personalities, and the hierarchy of biological organization from atom to organism. Chapters 2 through 4 explore carbohydrates, lipids, and proteins in depth their structures, their synthesis, their functions, and the molecular logic that connects structure to function in each case.

Chapter 5 focuses on enzymes the protein catalysts that make life's chemistry possible exploring kinetics, mechanism, and regulation in detail. Chapter 6 delves into nucleic acids: the chemistry of DNA and RNA, the double helix, the diversity of RNA molecules, and the packaging of DNA into chromosomes.

Chapters 7 and 8 trace the flow of biological information: how DNA is replicated with extraordinary fidelity, and how the genetic code is read and translated into protein sequences through the molecular machinery of transcription and translation.

Chapter 9 examines metabolism the integrated network of chemical reactions through which cells harvest energy from nutrients and use it to power all biological work, from glycolysis to the citric acid cycle to oxidative phosphorylation. Chapter 10 explores biomolecular communication the cell signaling pathways through which cells respond to their environment and coördinate their activities within multicellular organisms.

Chapter 11 brings the molecular perspective to bear on human disease and medicine exploring protein misfolding diseases, the molecular basis of cancer, drug design, monoclonal antibody therapy, and the CRISPR gene-editing revolution. Chapter 12 surveys the frontiers of biomolecular science: the omics revolution, synthetic biology, artificial intelligence in drug discovery, nanobiotechnology, and the ethical landscape of these powerful technologies.

Each chapter begins with a narrative introduction designed to place the chapter's content in its broader biological context to answer the question 'Why does this matter?' before asking 'What is this?' Each chapter concludes with a summary that consolidates the key concepts. Appendices provide reference material: the complete amino acid chart, the standard genetic code, metabolic pathway maps, a comprehensive glossary, and a guide to further reading.

IV.

A Note on Approach: Science as Story

Many excellent biochemistry textbooks exist. They are comprehensive, rigorously accurate, and invaluable reference works. This book aims to be something complementary rather than competing: a text that tells the story of biomolecules as the human and intellectual adventure that it is.

The molecules of life were not discovered in a vacuum. They were found by specific people, in specific historical moments, using specific tools often improvised, sometimes brilliant, occasionally lucky. Emil Fischer, working with primitive analytical chemistry at the end of the nineteenth century, deduced the stereochemical structures of the sugars through a feat of logical reasoning that stands as one of the greatest intellectual achievements in the history of chemistry. Rosalind Franklin, using X-ray crystallography of extraordinary technical quality, produced the images that revealed the geometry of the DNA double helix images whose significance was initially recognized not by her but by Watson and Crick. Kary Mullis, the inventor of the polymerase chain reaction, reportedly had the key insight while driving along a California highway at night, imagining the chemistry in his head.

These are not merely colorful anecdotes. They illustrate how science actually works not as the orderly accumulation of facts described in textbook introductions, but as a messy, competitive, creative, deeply human enterprise in which insight and luck, collaboration and conflict, play equal roles alongside technical skill and analytical rigor. Where the history of a discovery illuminates the science, this book tells that history. Where a metaphor or analogy makes a difficult concept vivid, this book uses it. Where the implications of a molecular discovery extend beyond the laboratory into medicine, ethics, or the philosophy of life, this book explores them.

At the same time, this book does not sacrifice scientific rigor for readability. Every concept presented here is consistent with current scientific understanding. Every mechanism described is based on experimental evidence. Every claim about the biological significance of a molecule or pathway reflects the consensus of the scientific community. The goal is not to simplify but to illuminate to make the full complexity of biomolecular science accessible without distorting it.

V.

For Whom This Book Is Written

This book is written primarily for students of biochemistry, molecular biology, cell biology, pharmacology, and medicine at the undergraduate and early postgraduate level students who have some background in general chemistry and biology and are ready to engage with biomolecules at depth. It assumes no prior knowledge of biochemistry, but it does assume intellectual curiosity and a willingness to engage with complex ideas.

It is also written for scientifically literate general readers physicians, nurses, science journalists, policy makers, and curious non-specialists who wish to understand what modern biomolecular science has revealed about the machinery of life, what it means for medicine and biotechnology, and what the great open questions are. The molecular revolution of the past century has changed our understanding of what life is and how it works in ways that are relevant to every thoughtful person, not only to scientists.

Finally, it is written for the student who has not yet chosen a field but who wants to understand why so many scientists find the molecular world endlessly fascinating. If you have wondered why cancer is so difficult to cure, or how CRISPR actually works, or what Alzheimer's disease looks like at the molecular level, or how a single fertilized cell becomes a trillion-celled organism this book is for you.

VI.

The Molecular Revolution and Its Consequences

We are living in an era defined by our growing ability to read, understand, and manipulate biological molecules with precision. The consequences of this ability are already transforming medicine, agriculture, energy, and materials science and the transformations are accelerating.

The Human Genome Project, completed in 2003, produced the first complete sequence of the human genome the full 3.2-billion-base-pair text of human heredity. Fifteen years later, the price of sequencing a human genome had fallen from three billion dollars to under five hundred, and clinical genomics the routine use of genome sequence data to guide diagnosis and treatment is becoming standard practice in major medical centers around the world. The identification of disease-causing mutations, the matching of cancer genotype to targeted therapy, the pharmacogenomic tailoring of drug doses to individual metabolic profiles all of these are now, or are rapidly becoming, routine clinical tools.

The development of CRISPR-Cas9 gene editing, announced in 2012, has made it possible to make precise changes to the genome of any organism cutting, inserting, deleting, or correcting specific sequences with a speed and simplicity that has democratized genetic engineering. The first CRISPR-based therapies were approved by the FDA in late 2023, for the treatment of sickle cell disease. Dozens more are in clinical trials. CRISPR is also being deployed in agriculture to produce disease-resistant crops, reduce food waste, and increase nutritional value and in basic research, where it has enabled the systematic functional annotation of genomes at a scale previously unimaginable.

Artificial intelligence is transforming structural biology and drug discovery. AlphaFold2, released by DeepMind in 2022, solved the long-standing protein folding problem predicting the three-dimensional structure of proteins from their amino acid sequence with near-experimental accuracy and has made predicted structures available for essentially all known proteins. This has transformed structural biology research and is accelerating structure-based drug design at an unprecedented pace.

Synthetic biology the engineering of biological systems with designed functions is producing organisms that manufacture pharmaceuticals, biofuels, biodegradable plastics, and industrial chemicals from renewable feedstocks. Cell-free protein synthesis, DNA data storage, protein nanocages for drug delivery, engineered bacteriophages for antibiotic-resistant infections the applications are proliferating faster than any single person can track.

All of these developments remarkable as they are rest on the foundational understanding of biomolecules that is the subject of this book. CRISPR works because we understand how DNA is recognized and cut by proteins. AlphaFold works because we understand the forces that govern protein folding. Gene therapy works because we understand how DNA is packaged and expressed. Targeted cancer drugs work because we understand the specific molecular mechanisms that drive cancer cell proliferation. In every case, the path from basic biomolecular knowledge to transformative application runs through exactly the kind of detailed understanding of structure and mechanism that this book aims to build.

VII.

An Invitation to Wonder

There is a particular kind of pleasure one that scientists know well but rarely advertise in understanding something deeply. Not merely knowing that the double helix carries genetic information, but understanding why the way the complementary base pairing of A with T and G with C is both the information storage mechanism and the copying mechanism, simultaneously elegant and functional, structure and function unified in a single molecular form. Not merely knowing that enzymes speed up reactions, but grasping the physical chemistry of transition state stabilization the way an active site creates a microenvironment that lowers the energy of the highest-energy point on the reaction pathway, making the impossible merely improbable and the improbable nearly instantaneous.

This kind of understanding deep, structural, mechanistic is what this book is designed to cultivate. It is harder than surface knowledge. It requires sustained attention, repeated encounters with difficult concepts, and a willingness to sit with confusion until clarity comes. But it is also incomparably more rewarding. Once you understand how a ribosome actually works the way the small subunit selects the correct tRNA through a kinetic proofreading mechanism that achieves extraordinary accuracy without sacrificing speed the ribosome becomes not just a fact but a marvel. Once you understand how a cell membrane regulates what enters and leaves the cell the precise architecture of ion channels, transporters, and receptors embedded in the lipid bilayer the cell becomes not a unit but a city.

The world is full of people who have learned, somewhere, that DNA is a double helix or that glucose is a sugar. This book aims to take you further to build the kind of molecular fluency that allows you not just to recite facts but to reason about biological problems from first principles, to read the scientific literature with comprehension, and to appreciate the molecular dimension of the medical and biotechnological questions that are shaping the twenty-first century.

It also aims to convey something that no amount of factual knowledge, on its own, can provide: a sense of the wonder that the molecular world inspires in those who look at it closely. The more deeply you understand the machinery of life, the more extraordinary it becomes. The more you learn about the precision and complexity of a single cell, the more remarkable it seems that such complexity could arise and that it could be understood.

This is the invitation of molecular biology: come and look closely at the smallest things, and find in them the largest questions. Come and learn the language that life speaks to itself. Come and join the conversation that has been going on between human curiosity and the molecular world for two centuries a conversation that, with each generation, reveals new wonders and opens new mysteries.

The molecules that matter are waiting. Turn the page, and begin.

— Abdus Salam
2026

CHAPTER 1

The Language of Life: An Introduction to Biomolecules

What Are Biomolecules and Why Do They Matter?

There is a quiet revolution happening inside you right now. Not a political uprising, not a social movement but something far more ancient, far more intimate, and incomprehensibly more complex. At this very moment, inside each of your approximately 37 trillion cells, millions of molecular machines are humming with activity. Proteins are folding into precise three-dimensional shapes. DNA is being read and copied. Sugars are being burned for energy. Membranes are flexing and signaling. Enzymes are catalyzing reactions at speeds that would make human engineers weep with envy.

This is the molecular world the world of biomolecules and it is the world this book is dedicated to exploring.

The word "biomolecule" might sound clinical or distant, but these are not abstract concepts locked away in the realm of specialists. Biomolecules are the stuff of you. They are what your food becomes after digestion. They are what makes a muscle contract, a neuron fire, a wound heal, a child develops from a single fertilized cell into a breathing, thinking, feeling human being. To understand biomolecules is to begin to understand life itself not as some mystical phenomenon beyond explanation, but as an elegant, deeply logical, and breathtakingly beautiful system of molecular interactions.

This opening chapter lays the foundation for everything that follows. We will explore what biomolecules are, where they come from chemically, and why the elements carbon, hydrogen, oxygen, nitrogen, phosphorus, and sulfur are the chosen building blocks of life. We will look at the role of water that deceptively simple molecule as the universal medium of biology. We will examine the chemical "handles" called functional groups that give biomolecules their diverse personalities. And we will take our first steps into the grand hierarchy that runs from atoms all the way up to living organisms.

1.1 What Is a Biomolecule?

A biomolecule, at its most fundamental level, is any molecule produced by a living organism that plays a role in biological processes. This definition, while accurate, barely scratches the surface of what these molecules actually do. A more meaningful way to appreciate biomolecules is to think of them as the vocabulary of a language the language that life uses to build, maintain, reproduce, and respond to its environment.

The study of biomolecules falls primarily within the discipline of biochemistry a field that emerged in the early twentieth century as a bridge between chemistry and biology. Before biochemistry, these two sciences operated largely in isolation. Chemists studied the properties of matter and the reactions between molecules. Biologists catalogued species, described anatomy, and theorized about heredity. It was only when investigators began asking the question "But how?" how does a muscle actually contract? how does food actually become energy? how does one cell become two? that the two disciplines were forced to merge.

The answer to all of those "how" questions turned out to be the same: molecules. Specifically, four great families of molecules that are universal to virtually all life on Earth. These are carbohydrates, lipids, proteins, and nucleic acids. These four classes are often called the macromolecules of life, and for good reason they are large, complex molecules that perform the core business of living.

But to understand why these particular molecules were selected by evolution over billions of years and countless chemical dead ends we must first appreciate the atomic raw materials that nature had available and chose to use.

1.2 The Chemistry of Life: Six Essential Elements

The periodic table contains 118 known elements, yet biology is remarkably almost stubbornly selective. Roughly 96% of the mass of a living organism is made up of just four elements: carbon, hydrogen, oxygen, and nitrogen. Add phosphorus and sulfur, and you have accounted for virtually all of biology's molecular architecture. Why these six? Why not silicon or iron or fluorine?

The answer lies in the unique properties of each element and how they combine.

Carbon is the undisputed king of biology. It is not merely useful it is indispensable. Carbon's genius lies in its electronic configuration: it has four valence electrons, which means it can form four covalent bonds simultaneously. This gives carbon an unmatched architectural versatility. It can bond to other carbons in straight chains, branching chains, or rings. It can form single, double, or triple bonds. It can attach to oxygen, nitrogen, hydrogen, sulfur, and phosphorus in almost limitless combinations. The result is a staggering diversity of carbon-based molecules biochemists estimate that the number of theoretically possible organic molecules runs into the billions, and living organisms have explored a remarkable fraction of this space.

Why not silicon, carbon's neighbor on the periodic table? Silicon also has four valence electrons, and this question is not a trivial one science fiction has long proposed silicon-based life. But silicon's bonds are weaker and less flexible than carbons. Silicon dioxide (sand) is a solid at room temperature, while carbon dioxide is a gas a critical difference. Life needs chemistry that can occur in aqueous solution, and carbon's compounds are far better suited to the wet, warm, dynamic environments of cells.

Hydrogen is the most abundant element in the universe, and in biology it serves as the universal glue. Hydrogen atoms bond to carbon to fill out molecular skeletons. They participate in hydrogen bonding a type of attractive interaction between molecules that is central to the structure of water, DNA, and proteins. Hydrogen is also shuffled between molecules during energy-transferring reactions, carried on the famous electron carriers NAD+ and FAD.

Oxygen brings electronegativity to the party a strong tendency to pull electrons toward itself. This property makes oxygen-containing functional groups highly reactive and excellent participants in the chemistry of metabolism. Oxygen forms double bonds with carbon to create carbonyl groups (as in sugars and amino acids) and is central to the reactions of cellular respiration, where it serves as the final electron acceptor in the great energy-harvesting cascade of the mitochondria.

Nitrogen is the defining element of amino acids and nucleic acids two of the most important classes of biological molecule. Nitrogen's ability to form three bonds and to bear a positive charge (as in the amino group, (H3+) makes it an ideal participant in the acid-base chemistry that governs protein structure and enzyme function. Nitrogen is also found in the nitrogenous bases of DNA and RNA adenine, guanine, cytosine, thymine, and uracil giving genetic molecules their information-storing capacity.

Phosphorus, though less abundant, plays an outsized role in biology. Phosphate groups ($PO4^{3-}$) form the backbone of DNA and RNA, link sugars together in certain polysaccharides, and most importantly make up adenosine triphosphate (ATP), the energy currency of all cells. The high-energy bonds of ATP are the key to how cells store and spend chemical energy.

Sulfur rounds out the six. Found in the amino acid's cysteine and methionine, sulfur can form disulfide bridges (–S–S–) between protein chains, helping to stabilize three-dimensional protein structures. It is also found in key metabolic molecules like coenzyme A, the shuttle that carries fatty acid fragments into cellular respiration.

Together, these six elements C, H, O, N, P, S form the molecular alphabet from which all of life is written.

1.3 The Miracle of Water: Biology's Universal Solvent

No discussion of biomolecules can proceed without first paying proper homage to water. H_2O is so familiar that we risk taking it entirely for granted. But from a chemist's perspective, water is one of the most extraordinary substances in the universe and life as we know it would be utterly impossible without its unique constellation of properties.

Water is a polar molecule. The oxygen atom, with its high electronegativity, pulls the shared electrons in the O–H bonds toward itself, giving the oxygen end a slight negative charge (δ–) and each hydrogen end a slight positive charge (δ+). This polarity means that water molecules are attracted to each other through hydrogen bonds the positive end of one molecule is attracted to the negative end of another. In liquid water at room temperature, each water molecule is engaged in an average of 3.4 hydrogen bonds simultaneously, creating a constantly shifting, dynamic network of molecular attractions.

This hydrogen bonding network is responsible for water's remarkable properties. Its boiling point (100°C) is extraordinarily high for a molecule of its size without hydrogen bonding, water would boil at around -80°C, and Earth's oceans would be vapor. Its high specific heat the amount of energy needed to raise its temperature means that water buffers temperature fluctuations, stabilizing the thermal environment of cells and of entire ecosystems. Its high heat of vaporization is why sweating cools us a relatively small amount of water, as it evaporates, carries away a large amount of heat.

Water is also the master solvent of biology. Its polarity allows it to dissolve ionic compounds (like salts) by surrounding individual ions and pulling them apart, and to solvate polar organic molecules by forming hydrogen bonds with their functional groups. Because biological reactions occur in solution, the ability of water to dissolve biomolecules is not a convenience it is an absolute necessity.

Not everything dissolves in water, and this fact, too, is biologically crucial. Nonpolar molecules molecules without significant charge separation, like the fatty hydrocarbon chains of lipids are hydrophobic (water-fearing). When placed in water, hydrophobic molecules are excluded from the hydrogen-bonding network of water and cluster together to minimize disruption. This hydrophobic effect is the thermodynamic force that drives the spontaneous formation of cell membranes the lipid bilayers that define the boundaries of cells and their internal compartments.

Water also participates directly in chemical reactions. Hydrolysis literally "water cutting" is the reaction by which polymers (large molecules built from repeating units) are broken down. When your body digests a protein, it is breaking peptide bonds through hydrolysis. When starch is broken down to glucose, water molecules cleave the glycosidic bonds. Water is not merely the medium of biology it is an active participant.

Finally, water's expansion upon freezing unique among small molecules means that ice floats on liquid water. This property ensures that lakes and rivers freeze from the top down, not the bottom up, preserving liquid water and aquatic life beneath the ice layer during winter. Had water behaved like most substances, freezing from the bottom, the world's aquatic ecosystems would have been catastrophically different and life's evolutionary history would have taken a radically different path.

1.4 Functional Groups: The Chemical Handles of Biomolecules

Biochemists often say that functional groups are to organic chemistry what accents are to a language they give molecules their distinctive character and determine how they interact with the world. A functional group is a specific arrangement of atoms within a molecule that confers characteristic chemical properties, regardless of the rest of the molecule's structure.

Understanding functional groups is not optional for understanding biochemistry it is foundational. The differences between a sugar and an amino acid, between a fat and a steroid, between an inhibitor and a substrate, can almost always be traced back to differences in their functional groups.

The hydroxyl group (–OH) is one of the most common functional groups in biomolecules. It consists of an oxygen atom bonded to a hydrogen atom. Hydroxyl groups make molecules polar and capable of hydrogen bonding, which dramatically increases their solubility in water. Sugars owe their water-loving nature largely to their multiple hydroxyl groups. Alcohols, by definition, contain a hydroxyl group, and many biologically important alcohols cholesterol, retinol (vitamin A), tocopherol (vitamin E) are central to physiology.

The carbonyl group (C=O) comes in two flavors depending on its position in a molecule. When the carbon of the carbonyl is at the end of a chain (bonded to a hydrogen), it forms an aldehyde. When the carbonyl carbon is in the middle of a chain (bonded to two other carbons), it forms a ketone. Both aldehydes and ketones are found in sugars glucose is an aldose (aldehyde sugar) while fructose is a ketose (ketone sugar). Carbonyl groups are also found in amino acids, peptide bonds, and numerous metabolic intermediates.

The carboxyl group (–COOH) is the defining group of organic acids, and it is profoundly important in biology. It consists of a carbon double-bonded to an oxygen and single-bonded to a hydroxyl group. Under physiological conditions, carboxyl groups tend to lose their hydrogen ion (H+), carrying a negative charge. Amino acids have a carboxyl group at one end of their structure, and fatty acids are essentially long hydrocarbon chains terminated by a carboxyl group.

The amino group ($-NH_2$) is the defining group of amines, and in biological context it is most famously found in amino acids (hence the name). Amino groups are basic they tend to accept a hydrogen ion from solution, becoming $-NH_3$+ and carrying a positive charge. This acid-base behavior of amino and carboxyl groups is what gives amino acids their buffering capacity and their ability to form the peptide bonds that link them into proteins.

The phosphate group ($-PO_4^{2-}$) deserves special mention for its extraordinary role in biology. Phosphate groups carry two negative charges under physiological conditions, making any molecule that contains one highly polar and charged. More importantly, phosphate groups can form high-energy bonds with themselves as in the two "energy-rich" bonds of ATP and with biological molecules, serving as molecular switches that turn proteins on or off through a process called phosphorylation.

The sulfhydryl group (–SH), found in the amino acid cysteine, is the source of that amino acid's remarkable ability to form disulfide bridges. Two cysteine sulfhydryl groups can be oxidized to form a covalent –S–S– bond, which acts as a molecular staple holding regions of a protein together. This is how the three-dimensional structure of many proteins including insulin, antibodies, and keratin (the protein of hair and nails) is maintained.

1.5 From Atoms to Organisms: Levels of Biological Organization

One of the most awe-inspiring aspects of biology is the seamless way in which the very small gives rise to the very large. There is no sharp boundary, no magical transition, between chemistry and life only an extraordinary elaboration of molecular complexity, layer upon layer, until something breathes and moves and thinks.

The simplest level is that of atoms the individual carbon, hydrogen, oxygen, nitrogen, phosphorus, and sulfur atoms we discussed earlier. These atoms are not in themselves alive. They obey the same laws of physics and chemistry whether they are part of a living cell or a lump of coal.

The next level is that of small molecules the building blocks of biology. Glucose (a simple sugar), glycerol (a fat component), single amino acids, individual nucleotides these are small enough to be defined by precise chemical formulas and to be synthesized in a laboratory. They are the monomers: the single units from which larger structures are built.

Macromolecules represent the third level. These are the polymers large molecules built by linking many monomers together through condensation reactions (reactions that release water). A single protein molecule may contain hundreds or thousands of amino acid monomers linked in a precise sequence. A DNA molecule can contain billions of nucleotide monomers arranged in the particular sequence that constitutes a gene. At this level, the concept of "information" begins to emerge the sequence of monomers in a macromolecule carries biological meaning.

Supramolecular assemblies are formed when multiple macromolecules come together through non-covalent interactions. Ribosomes the molecular machines that synthesize proteins are assemblies of ribosomal RNA and proteins. Cell membranes are assemblies of lipid molecules, embedded proteins, and carbohydrate chains. Chromatin the packaging of DNA in the nucleus is an assembly of DNA and histone proteins. These assemblies are not held together by the covalent bonds of chemistry but by weaker, reversible interactions: hydrogen bonds, ionic attractions, hydrophobic forces, and van der Waals forces.

Organelles represent the next step: membrane-bound compartments within the cell, each specialized for particular functions. The mitochondrion, with its elaborate internal membrane systems, is the site of ATP synthesis. The endoplasmic reticulum is the site of protein processing and lipid synthesis. The Golgi apparatus modifies and sorts proteins for delivery to their correct destinations.

Then comes the cell itself the basic unit of life. A cell is the smallest entity that can be said to be alive in any meaningful sense. It contains all the machinery necessary for metabolism, growth, response to stimuli, and reproduction. From a single cell, an entire organism can develop, given the right instructions encoded in its DNA.

And from collections of cells tissues, organs, organ systems we arrive finally at the organism: the level at which all this molecular complexity manifests as something we can see, touch, and talk to.

This hierarchy atom, molecule, macromolecule, supramolecular assembly, organelle, cell, tissue, organ, organism is not just an organizational convenience. It is the actual architecture of biology. And the foundation of every single level is molecular. This is why molecules matter.

1.6 Historical Milestones: The Making of Biochemistry

The history of biochemistry is a story of persistent curiosity triumphing over the apparent inscrutability of life. For most of human history, the workings of the living body were attributed to vital forces mysterious essences that were thought to animate matter and make it alive. This concept, known as vitalism, held that life was fundamentally different from non-life, governed by principles that chemistry could never reach.

The first decisive blow against vitalism was struck in 1828 by Friedrich Wöhler, a German chemist who synthesized urea a compound found in urine and therefore considered a "biological" substance from purely inorganic starting materials. Wöhler's synthesis demonstrated that there was no magical boundary between the chemistry of the living and the non-living. If urea could be made in a flask, then perhaps the other molecules of life could be understood and eventually replicated by the chemist's art.

The following decades saw explosive progress. Louis Pasteur demonstrated that fermentation was caused by living microorganisms' yeasts rather than purely chemical processes. But in 1897, Eduard Buchner showed that cell-free extracts of yeast could ferment sugars just as effectively as intact yeast cells. The active agents, it turned out, were proteins the class of molecules we now call enzymes. Life's chemistry did not require the intact cell; it required the right molecules.

The early twentieth century brought the first serious analyses of biological macromolecules. Emil Fischer worked out the basic chemistry of amino acids and sugars, establishing the concepts of peptide bonds and glycosidic bonds. Frederick Sanger, in the 1950s, became the first person to determine the complete amino acid sequence of a protein insulin proving that proteins had precise, definite structures.

The discovery of DNA's role as the genetic material came in stages. Frederick Griffith's experiments in 1928 showed that some "transforming principle" could convert harmless bacteria into lethal ones. In 1944, Avery, MacLeod, and McCarty identified that transforming principle as DNA. And then, in 1953, James Watson and Francis Crick proposed the double helix model of DNA structure arguably the most important scientific discovery of the twentieth century building on X-ray diffraction data produced by Rosalind Franklin and Raymond Gosling.

The double helix immediately suggested how genetic information is stored and copied, launching the molecular biology revolution. The genetic code the rules by which DNA sequences are translated into protein sequences was cracked in the 1960s through the combined efforts of Marshall Nirenberg, Har Gobind Khorana, and others. The polymerase chain reaction (PCR), invented by Kary Mullis in 1983, made it possible to amplify specific DNA sequences with extraordinary precision. Recombinant DNA technology, gene sequencing, genomics, proteomics, and finally CRISPR-Cas9 gene editing have all flowed from this foundational understanding of biomolecules.

Each of these milestones represents a moment when human ingenuity found a way to speak the language of life to read it, and eventually, to write it. This book is an invitation to learn that language.

Chapter Summary

Life is built from molecules, and understanding life requires understanding these molecules. Six elements carbon, hydrogen, oxygen, nitrogen, phosphorus, and sulfur form the chemical backbone of all biomolecules. Carbon's unique ability to form four covalent bonds in diverse arrangements makes it the architectural foundation of biological complexity.

Water, with its polarity and capacity for hydrogen bonding, creates the medium in which all biology unfolds. Its extraordinary properties high boiling point, high specific heat, universal solvent capacity, and the hydrophobic effect it generates are not coincidences of nature but the very conditions that made life possible on Earth.

Functional groups hydroxyl, carbonyl, carboxyl, amino, phosphate, and sulfhydryl are the chemical "handles" that give biomolecules their distinct properties and reactivities. These groups determine solubility, charge, reactivity, and the types of bonds that can form between molecules.

The four major classes of biomolecules carbohydrates, lipids, proteins, and nucleic acids are each explored in depth in the chapters that follow. Together, they constitute the molecular machinery of all life. The history of biochemistry, from Wöhler's synthesis of urea to the CRISPR revolution, is the story of humanity gradually learning to read and understand this machinery.

In the chapters ahead, we will explore each class of biomolecule in detail their structures, their functions, and their roles in the grand project of life. We begin, as life itself does in terms of energy, with carbohydrates.

CHAPTER 2

Carbohydrates: The Fuel and Framework of Life

Structure, Classification, and Metabolic Roles

Imagine holding a single grain of table sugar between your fingers. It seems almost impossibly simple a tiny white crystal, barely visible, without smell or color. Yet that crystal contains approximately 10^{21} molecules of sucrose, each one a precisely structured combination of two smaller sugar molecules locked together by a covalent bond. And when that sucrose enters your body, it embarks on a journey of extraordinary chemical transformation broken apart, reconfigured, burned for energy, built into storage polymers, attached to proteins, incorporated into cell membranes, and used to carry information between cells.

Carbohydrates are perhaps the most misunderstood of the four major biomolecule classes. In popular culture, "carbs" have been simultaneously celebrated and vilified praised by athletes as performance fuel and demonized by dieters as the enemy of leanness. This cultural conversation, though not without some biochemical basis, dramatically understates the biological diversity and importance of this molecule class. Carbohydrates are not just bread and pasta. They are the structural material of plant cell walls. They are the informational tags on the surfaces of your red blood cells that determine your blood type. They are the gels in your connective tissue. They are the fuel for your brain's insatiable demand for glucose. They are everywhere, doing everything.

This chapter explores the full remarkable world of carbohydrates from the simplest single sugars to the vast, complex polysaccharides that build cellulose trees and store energy in your liver. Along the way, we will encounter the chemical logic of ring formation, the critical concept of anomers, the chemistry of the glycosidic bond, and the profound biological consequences of seemingly small structural differences.

2.1 What Are Carbohydrates? The Basic Chemical Definition

The word "carbohydrate" literally means "carbon hydrate" a historical artifact from the early days of organic chemistry, when these molecules were believed to be simple hydrates of carbon. The general formula $Cn(H_2O)$ n seemed to fit: glucose is $C_6H_{12}O_6$, which can be written as $C_6(H_2O)_6$. We now know this formula is not really accurate for all carbohydrates, and that the "hydrate" idea is chemically misleading, but the name has stuck.

A more accurate chemical definition is this: carbohydrates are polyhydroxy aldehydes or polyhydroxy ketones molecules with multiple hydroxyl (–OH) groups and either an aldehyde (–CHO) or a ketone (C=O) functional group. This definition captures what is essential about the chemistry of simple sugars. The multiple hydroxyl groups make them highly soluble in water and capable of extensive hydrogen bonding. The aldehyde or ketone group makes them chemically reactive and capable of participating in ring formation and bond-forming reactions.

Carbohydrates are classified primarily by the number of sugar units they contain. Monosaccharides are the simplest single sugar units that cannot be further hydrolyzed. Disaccharides consist of two monosaccharides joined by a glycosidic bond. Oligosaccharides contain a small number (typically 3–10) of monosaccharide units. And polysaccharides are long chains of many monosaccharide units sometimes thousands linked together into complex, often branched structures.

This hierarchical classification mirrors the general principle of biological macromolecules: simple monomers, linked by specific bonds, give rise to polymers of extraordinary structural and functional diversity.

2.2 Monosaccharides: The Sweet Simplicity of Single Sugars

Monosaccharides are the foundational vocabulary of carbohydrate chemistry. They are the monomers from which all larger carbohydrates are built, and they are themselves biologically active in important ways. The most biologically important monosaccharides are the hexoses six-carbon sugar among which glucose, fructose, and galactose are the leading players.

Glucose ($C_6H_{12}O_6$) is arguably the most important single molecule in all of biology. It is the preferred fuel of the brain, the immediate product of photosynthesis, the starting material of glycolysis, and the monomer of the most abundant organic molecule on Earth cellulose. When we speak of blood sugar, we mean blood glucose. When we speak of blood sugar regulation, we mean the intricate hormonal dance that keeps glucose concentration in the blood within a narrow, life-sustaining range.

Fructose is an isomer of glucose it has the same molecular formula but a different arrangement of atoms. Where glucose has an aldehyde group at carbon-1 (making it an aldose), fructose has a ketone group at carbon-2 (making it a ketose). This seemingly small difference has significant consequences: fructose is sweeter than glucose (it is the sugar that makes fruit taste sweet) and it enters metabolic pathways at different points. Excessive fructose consumption particularly from high-fructose corn syrup in processed foods has been associated with metabolic dysfunction, including elevated triglycerides and increased risk of non-alcoholic fatty liver disease.

Galactose is another glucose isomer, differing from glucose only in the orientation of the hydroxyl group at carbon-4. This tiny structural difference a single –OH pointing in a different direction completely changes how galactose is recognized by enzymes and receptors. Galactose is found combined with glucose in lactose (milk sugar) and is an important component of glycoproteins and glycolipids on cell surfaces. People with galactosemia, a genetic condition in which an enzyme needed to metabolize galactose is defective, cannot tolerate milk and must avoid it from birth.

Monosaccharides can be classified not only by the functional group they carry (aldose vs. ketose) but also by the number of carbons in their backbone. Trioses (3 carbons), tetroses (4 carbons), pentoses (5 carbons), hexoses (6 carbons), and heptoses

(7 carbons) all occur biologically. The pentoses ribose and deoxyribose are of particular importance as the sugar components of RNA and DNA, respectively. The difference between them is one oxygen atom: deoxyribose lacks the hydroxyl group at carbon-2 that ribose carries. As we will see in Chapter 6, this single difference has profound implications for the stability and function of these nucleic acids.

One of the most important concepts in monosaccharide chemistry is the Fischer projection a two-dimensional representation of sugar structures that shows the spatial arrangement of groups around each carbon. The designation D or L before a sugar's name refers to the absolute configuration at the highest-numbered chiral carbon (the carbon immediately above the CH_2OH group in a Fischer projection). Virtually all biologically occurring sugars are of the D configuration. L-sugars do exist and can be synthesized in the lab, but they are generally not recognized by the enzymes of biological metabolism a beautiful example of the exquisite stereochemical specificity of biochemistry.

2.3 Ring Forms and Anomers: When Chemistry Goes in Circles

Here is where carbohydrate chemistry becomes genuinely surprising. In solution which is where biology happens glucose does not actually exist primarily as an open-chain molecule with a free aldehyde group. Instead, it spontaneously undergoes intramolecular cyclization: the aldehyde at carbon-1 reacts with the hydroxyl group at carbon-5, forming a six-membered ring called a pyranose ring (named after the heterocyclic compound pyran, which it resembles).

This cyclization creates a new chiral center at carbon-1, called the anomeric carbon. The hydroxyl group at this carbon can point either downward (below the plane of the ring, designated α) or upward (above the plane of the ring, designated β). These two forms are called anomers, and they are not merely academic distinctions they have profoundly different biological consequences.

In α-D-glucose, the hydroxyl group at carbon-1 is on the same side as the ring. In β-D-glucose, it is on the opposite side. In solution, glucose interconverts between the α and β forms through the open-chain intermediate, a process called mutarotation. At equilibrium in aqueous solution, the mixture contains about 36% α-D-glucose, 64% β-D-glucose, and less than 0.02% open-chain form.

Why does this matter? Because the enzymes that use glucose are exquisitely sensitive to its anomeric form. Glycogen phosphorylase, the enzyme that breaks down glycogen to release glucose-1-phosphate, acts specifically on α-glucosidic linkages. Cellulase enzymes, which break down cellulose, act on β-glucosidic linkages. The glycosidic bonds that join monosaccharides into polymers discussed in the next section specify their anomeric configuration, and this specification completely determines the three-dimensional structure and properties of the resulting polysaccharide.

The difference between starch and cellulose one digestible, one not; one soft, one rigid; one energy reserve, one structural material comes down entirely to the anomeric configuration of a single bond: α versus β.

2.4 Disaccharides: When Two Sugars Become One

When two monosaccharides join together, they form a disaccharide through a condensation reaction: the hydroxyl group on one sugar reacts with the anomeric hydroxyl of another, releasing a water molecule and forming a covalent bond called a glycosidic bond. The resulting disaccharide retains one free anomeric carbon (unless both anomeric carbons participated in the bond, as in the case of sucrose) and can in principle be hydrolyzed back to its component monosaccharides.

Sucrose — ordinary table sugar is the disaccharide most familiar to humans, and it is one of the most abundant organic molecules on Earth, produced by plants in enormous quantities for transport of carbohydrate energy from leaves to other tissues. Sucrose consists of glucose and fructose joined by a bond between both of their anomeric carbons (α-1, β-2 glycosidic bond). This unusual linkage means that sucrose has no free anomeric carbon, making it a non-reducing sugar it cannot reduce oxidizing agents in the classic chemical tests for sugars. It also means that sucrose cannot mutarotate and that both of its component sugars are "committed" their anomeric positions are locked.

Lactose milk sugar is the disaccharide of galactose and glucose, linked by a β (1→4) glycosidic bond. It is the primary carbohydrate of mammalian milk and is the reason that newborn mammals can digest milk as their primary food source. The enzyme lactase, produced in the small intestinal epithelium, cleaves lactose into its component sugars for absorption. Most humans produce abundant lactase as infants but gradually reduce production after weaning. The persistence of lactase activity into adulthood a condition called lactase persistence is a genetic adaptation that evolved independently in several human populations with long traditions of cattle herding and dairy farming. Its distribution today maps almost perfectly onto the historical geography of pastoral cultures.

Maltose, the disaccharide of two glucose units joined by an α (1→4) bond, is produced when starch is partially digested by amylase enzymes. It is found in germinating grain seeds and gives malt beverages their characteristic flavor. Maltose is a reducing sugar it retains one free anomeric carbon and can be further hydrolyzed by the enzyme maltase to yield two glucose molecules.

Trehalose, a disaccharide of two glucose units joined between both anomeric carbons, is found in many organisms that can survive extreme dehydration: insects, crustaceans, nematodes, and certain plants called resurrection plants can withstand complete desiccation and then rehydrate fully when water becomes available. Trehalose appears to protect cellular membranes and proteins during dehydration by forming a glassy matrix around them, replacing the water molecules that normally interact with their surfaces.

2.5 Polysaccharides: The Great Carbohydrate Polymers

When monosaccharides are linked not in pairs but in chains of dozens, hundreds, or even thousands, the result is a polysaccharide a macromolecule of carbohydrate chemistry. Polysaccharides are the most abundant organic molecules on Earth, and their diversity of structure and function is remarkable.

Starch is the primary energy storage polysaccharide of plants. It exists in two forms: amylose and amylopectin. Amylose is an essentially linear chain of glucose units linked by α (1→4) bonds, which causes it to adopt a helical shape in solution. Amylopectin has the same α (1→4) backbone but with α (1→6) branches occurring approximately every 24–30 glucose units. These branches increase the molecule's solubility and create multiple chain ends from which glucose can be rapidly released when energy is needed.

When you eat a potato, a bowl of rice, or a piece of bread, you are primarily consuming starch. The enzyme salivary amylase begins starch digestion in your mouth this is why bread starts to taste slightly sweet as you chew it and pancreatic amylase completes digestion in the small intestine, ultimately releasing glucose for absorption into the bloodstream.

Glycogen is the animal analog of starch the primary carbohydrate energy reserve of animal cells. It is structurally similar to amylopectin but even more highly branched, with branch points occurring approximately every 8–12 glucose units. This extreme branching creates a spherical, tree-like molecule of enormous size and surface area. The human liver stores approximately 100 grams of glycogen, which can be rapidly mobilized to maintain blood glucose between meals. Muscles store an additional 300–400 grams, which is used locally during exercise.

Cellulose is the world's most abundant organic molecule. It is the principal structural component of plant cell walls, and its production by photosynthetic organisms is estimated at over 100 billion metric tons per year making it the overwhelmingly dominant biological polymer on Earth. Cellulose, like starch, is made entirely from glucose — but the glucose units are joined by β (1→4) bonds rather than α (1→4) bonds. This single difference in anomeric configuration changes everything. The β linkage allows individual glucose units to adopt a flat, extended conformation, and adjacent chains can hydrogen-bond to each other along their entire lengths, creating rigid, rope-like microfibrils of extraordinary tensile strength.

Humans cannot digest cellulose because we lack the enzyme cellulase, which breaks β (1→4) bonds. The cellulose in plant foods passes through our digestive system largely intact this is what we call dietary fiber. But many bacteria, fungi, and protists can produce cellulase, and these organisms are responsible for the decomposition of plant material worldwide. Termites harbor cellulase-producing microorganisms in their guts, which is how they can derive nutrition from wood.

Chitin is a structural polysaccharide found in the exoskeletons of arthropods (insects, crustaceans, spiders) and in the cell walls of fungi. It is chemically similar to cellulose but with one important modification: the hydroxyl group at carbon-2 of each glucose unit is replaced by an acetylamino group ($-NHCOCH_3$), making the monomer N-acetylglucosamine. The β (1→4) linkages between these modified glucose units give chitin the same flat, extended chain structure as cellulose, and the hydrogen bonding between chains creates similar rigidity and strength. After cellulose, chitin is the second most abundant organic polymer on Earth.

2.6 Carbohydrates in Signaling: Glycoproteins and Glycolipids

Perhaps the most underappreciated role of carbohydrates in biology is their function as molecular information tags. The surfaces of virtually all animal cells are coated with a rich forest of carbohydrate chains the glycocalyx attached to proteins (glycoproteins) and lipids (glycolipids) of the cell membrane. This carbohydrate coat is the cell's identification badge, the interface through which it communicates with the outside world.

Glycoproteins are proteins with oligosaccharide chains covalently attached at specific amino acid residues. The sugars in these chains are linked to asparagine (N-linked glycosylation) or to serine/threonine (O-linked glycosylation). The carbohydrate portions of glycoproteins serve many functions: they aid in the proper folding of the protein in the endoplasmic reticulum, protect against proteolytic degradation, mediate cell-cell recognition, and participate in the binding of hormones, growth factors, and pathogens to cell surfaces.

Blood type is perhaps the most familiar example of carbohydrate-mediated cell recognition. The ABO blood group system is determined not by proteins but by carbohydrates specifically, by oligosaccharide chains attached to glycolipids and glycoproteins on the surface of red blood cells. Type A individuals carry a terminal N-acetyl galactosamine residue. Type B individuals carry a terminal galactose. Type AB individuals carry both. Type O individuals have neither. Your immune system is sensitized to recognize these sugars as "self" and to generate antibodies against the "foreign" sugars which is why giving someone the wrong blood type triggers a potentially fatal immune reaction.

This carbohydrate-based cell recognition system is exploited not only by your own immune system but also by pathogens. Many viruses, bacteria, and toxins gain entry to human cells by binding to specific carbohydrate structures on the cell surface. The influenza virus, for example, binds to sialic acid residues on glycoproteins of respiratory epithelial cells. The HIV virus binds to CD4 glycoprotein (which has carbohydrate chains) on helper T cells.

The ability to block these carbohydrate-receptor interactions is an active area of antiviral and antibacterial drug research.

Proteoglycans a special class of glycoprotein in which the carbohydrate content is extremely high form the gel-like matrix of connective tissue. Hyaluronic acid, chondroitin sulfate, and heparin sulfate are examples of the glycosaminoglycan (GAG) chains found in proteoglycans. These molecules are responsible for the elasticity of cartilage, the lubrication of joints, the hydration of the vitreous humor of the eye, and the anticoagulant activity of blood-contacting surfaces. In short, they are the molecular shock absorbers and lubricants of the body.

Chapter Summary

Carbohydrates are a structurally and functionally diverse class of biomolecules whose common thread is a backbone of carbon atoms bearing hydroxyl groups and either an aldehyde or a ketone. Monosaccharides are the monomeric units, existing in open-chain and ring (pyranose or furanose) forms. The anomeric carbon created during ring formation gives rise to α and β anomers a distinction with profound consequences for polymer structure and digestibility.

Disaccharides sucrose, lactose, maltose link pairs of monosaccharides through glycosidic bonds. Polysaccharides starch, glycogen, cellulose, chitin — are the great carbohydrate polymers, serving as energy stores and structural materials. The difference between the digestible starch and the indigestible cellulose comes down to a single bond angle: α versus β glycosidic linkage.

Beyond energy and structure, carbohydrates serve as the molecular identity tags of cells. The glycocalyx the carbohydrate coat of animal cells mediates cell recognition, immune function, blood typing, and pathogen entry. Glycoproteins and glycolipids are the molecular alphabet by which cells communicate with each other and with the external world.

In the next chapter, we turn to lipids the hydrophobic molecules that define the boundaries of cells, store energy in concentrated form, and carry some of the most potent biological signals in the body.

CHAPTER 3

Lipids: Membranes, Energy, and Signaling Molecules

The Diverse World of Hydrophobic Biomolecules

Of the four great classes of biomolecules, lipids are the most chemically heterogeneous. Unlike carbohydrates, proteins, and nucleic acids — which can each be defined by a characteristic covalent backbone lipids are defined not by structure but by behavior: they are the biomolecules that are insoluble in water but soluble in non-polar organic solvents. This definition unites an extraordinarily diverse collection of molecules: the fats stored in your adipose tissue, the phospholipids that form every cell membrane in your body, the cholesterol that regulates membrane fluidity, the steroid hormones that govern development and metabolism, the fat-soluble vitamins, the insulating wax coatings of leaves and skin, and the powerful lipid signaling molecules that

mediate inflammation and pain.

This diversity is lipidology's greatest challenge and its greatest fascination. There is no single "lipid structure" to memorize, no universal lipid backbone. Instead, there is a family of molecules united by hydrophobicity by the shared property of being poorly soluble in water and by the extraordinary variety of biological roles that this hydrophobicity enables.

The key to understanding this diversity is the fatty acid the hydrocarbon chain that forms the non-polar tail of most lipid molecules. Almost every major lipid class is built from, contains, or is related to fatty acid chains. Starting with fatty acids, we can build triglycerides (fats), phospholipids (membranes), and waxes. From a sterol precursor derived from fatty acid synthesis, we can build cholesterol, steroid hormones, bile acids, and vitamin D. Once you understand the fatty acid, the rest of lipid biochemistry becomes navigable.

3.1 Fatty Acids: The Molecular Building Blocks of Lipids

A fatty acid is a carboxylic acid with a long hydrocarbon tail. The carboxyl group (–COOH) at one end is polar and ionized at physiological pH (bearing a negative charge as $-COO^-$). The hydrocarbon tail a chain of carbon and hydrogen atoms is non-polar and hydrophobic. This split personality is the key to fatty acid function: the polar head can interact with water, while the non-polar tail avoids it.

Fatty acids are characterized by two primary properties: chain length and degree of saturation. Most naturally occurring fatty acids have even numbers of carbons a consequence of their biosynthesis, which occurs two carbons at a time and chain lengths between 12 and 20 carbons are most common in biology.

Saturated fatty acids have no double bonds in their hydrocarbon chains. The carbon atoms are "saturated" with hydrogen atoms they cannot accept any more without breaking the chain. Saturated fatty acids are straight and relatively rigid, and this allows individual molecules to pack tightly together through van der Waals forces. This tight packing is why saturated fats (found in animal products like butter, lard, and beef fat) are solid at room temperature. Palmitic acid (16 carbons, no double bonds) and stearic acid (18 carbons, no double bonds) are the most common saturated fatty acids in human biology.

Unsaturated fatty acids have one or more double bonds in their hydrocarbon chains. Each double bond introduces a bend or kink in the chain, preventing tight packing and lowering the melting point. Monounsaturated fatty acids have a single double bond. Oleic acid (18 carbons, one double bond at the 9th carbon position) is the most abundant fatty acid in the human body and in olive oil, and it is associated with the cardiovascular benefits of the Mediterranean diet.

Polyunsaturated fatty acids (PUFAs) have two or more double bonds. Linoleic acid (18 carbons, two double bonds) and α-linolenic acid (18 carbons, three double bonds) are considered essential fatty acids they cannot be synthesized by the human body and must be obtained from the diet. From linoleic acid, the body can synthesize the omega-6 fatty acids (arachidonic acid and others). From α-linolenic acid, it can synthesize the omega-3 fatty acids, including EPA (eicosatetraenoic acid) and DHA (docosahexaenoic acid) the fatty acids particularly abundant in fatty fish and linked to cardiovascular and neurological health.

The position and geometry of double bonds in unsaturated fatty acids have important biological consequences. Nearly all naturally occurring double bonds in biological fatty acids are in the cis configuration the hydrocarbon chain bends back on itself at the double bond, creating the characteristic kink. Trans fatty acids, by contrast, have their hydrogens on opposite sides of the double bond, which allows the chain to remain more linear and to pack more tightly more like a saturated fat. Trans fats occur naturally in small amounts in ruminant animal products, but they are primarily found in partially hydrogenated vegetable oils industrial fats created by a chemical process that introduces trans double bonds. Trans fats have been clearly linked to increased cardiovascular disease risk, and many countries have now banned or severely restricted their use in food production.

3.2 Triglycerides: The Body's Premier Energy Reserve

Triglycerides (also called triacylglycerols) are the principal form in which fatty acids are stored in the body. Structurally, a triglyceride consists of one glycerol molecule a three-carbon alcohol with a hydroxyl group on each carbon to which three fatty acid chains are attached through ester bonds. The process of forming these ester bonds, like all condensation reactions in biology, releases one water molecule per bond formed.

The result is a large, highly non-polar molecule that packs into dense, anhydrous (water-free) droplets in specialized fat storage cells called adipocytes. This anhydrous packing is extremely important from an energy perspective. Fats store about 9 kilocalories of energy per gram more than twice the 4 kilocalories per gram stored by carbohydrates or proteins. This superior energy density arises from the highly reduced state of the carbon atoms in fatty acid chains: they carry many hydrogen atoms, and these can be oxidized (stripped of electrons) to generate ATP with great efficiency.

For a person of average body weight, the triglyceride reserves in adipose tissue represent approximately 100,000–150,000 kilocalories of stored energy enough to survive weeks without food. By contrast, the glycogen reserves of the liver and muscles represent only about 1,500 kilocalories enough for only about 24 hours of fasting. This is why prolonged fasting ultimately depends on fat oxidation rather than glycogen breakdown.

Dietary triglycerides the fats in olive oil, beef, butter, and nuts are digested in the small intestine through the action of pancreatic lipase, an enzyme that cleaves fatty acids from the glycerol backbone. The released fatty acids and monoglycerides are packaged into micelles (tiny lipid droplets surrounded by bile salts) and absorbed by intestinal epithelial cells. Inside these cells, triglycerides are reassembled and packaged into chylomicrons large lipid-protein particles that enter the lymphatic system and ultimately the bloodstream, where they deliver fatty acids to tissues throughout the body.

Brown adipose tissue (BAT) deserves special mention as a specialized form of fat that exists not to store energy but to burn it specifically, to generate heat. Brown fat is rich in mitochondria (giving it its characteristic dark color) and expresses a unique protein called uncoupling protein 1 (UCP1), which allows the energy released by fat oxidation to dissipate as heat rather than being captured in ATP. This thermogenic activity is critical for maintaining body temperature in newborns and in hibernating animals. Recent discoveries have shown that adult humans also possess significant amounts of brown adipose tissue, and its activation by cold exposure or certain hormones is an active area of research for obesity treatment.

3.3 Phospholipids and the Lipid Bilayer: The Foundation of Membranes

If there is one structural concept in all of cell biology that stands above all others in elegance and importance, it is the lipid bilayer the self-assembling, fluid, selectively permeable membrane that defines the boundary of every cell and every intracellular compartment. And at the heart of the lipid bilayer is the phospholipid.

A phospholipid is structurally similar to a triglyceride, but with a crucial difference: one of the three fatty acid chains is replaced by a phosphate group bearing a polar or charged head group. The result is a molecule with a distinct amphipathic character it has both a non-polar region (the two fatty acid tails) and a polar region (the phosphate head group). This split personality is the key to everything.

The most common phospholipids in animal cell membranes include phosphatidylcholine (PC), phosphatidylethanolamine (PE), phosphatidylserine (PS), and phosphatidylinositol (PI). Each has the same basic glycerophospholipid backbone but a different head group attached to the phosphate. The head groups vary in charge, size, and chemical reactivity, and these differences determine the specific functions of each phospholipid type.

When phospholipids are placed in water, their amphipathic nature drives spontaneous self-assembly. The hydrophobic tails cluster together to avoid contact with water, while the hydrophilic head groups remain exposed to the aqueous environment on both sides. The thermodynamically most stable arrangement the one that minimizes the exposure of hydrophobic surfaces to water is the bilayer: two sheets of phospholipids arranged tail-to-tail, with the head groups facing outward into the aqueous environment on both sides.

This bilayer is not rigid. It is a fluid, dynamic structure in which individual phospholipid molecules move rapidly within the plane of the membrane a phenomenon described by the fluid mosaic model, proposed by Singer and Nicholson in 1972. In this model, the lipid bilayer acts as a two-dimensional fluid in which proteins float and move, like icebergs in a sea of lipid. Phospholipids can rotate rapidly around their long axis and diffuse laterally (parallel to the membrane surface) at rates of several micrometers per second. This lateral mobility allows the membrane to be flexible, to allow the fusion of vesicles, and to enable the lateral diffusion of membrane proteins to sites of cellular activity.

The fluidity of the membrane is regulated by the composition of the fatty acid chains in the phospholipids. Unsaturated fatty acids, with their kinks, disrupt regular packing and increase fluidity. Saturated fatty acids promote tighter packing and reduce fluidity. Organisms that must function at variable temperatures such as fish in cold water adjust the proportion of unsaturated fatty acids in their membranes to maintain appropriate fluidity: a process called homeoviscous adaptation.

3.4 Cholesterol: Master Regulator of Membrane Properties

Cholesterol is perhaps the most famous and most misunderstood lipid molecule in biology. In popular consciousness, cholesterol is associated primarily with heart disease and dietary fat. In biological reality, it is an absolutely essential molecule without which animal cells cannot survive, a master regulator of membrane fluidity, and the precursor to some of the most important signaling molecules in the body.

Cholesterol is a sterol a member of the steroid family of lipids characterized by a rigid four-ring hydrocarbon skeleton (three six-membered rings and one five-membered ring fused together) with various functional groups and side chains attached. It has a single hydroxyl group at one end (making that end slightly polar) and an entirely non-polar hydrocarbon skeleton and tail. When inserted into a phospholipid bilayer, cholesterol tucks itself between phospholipid molecules with its hydroxyl group near the polar head groups and its rigid ring system extending into the hydrophobic core of the membrane.

The effect of cholesterol on membrane fluidity is complex and context-dependent. At high temperatures, cholesterol reduces fluidity by interacting with and immobilizing the fatty acid tails of neighboring phospholipids. At low temperatures, cholesterol interferes with the tight packing of phospholipid tails and prevents the membrane from crystallizing into a gel-like state. The net effect is that cholesterol acts as a membrane fluidity buffer smoothing out the extremes of temperature-dependent changes. This is one reason that cells tightly regulate their cholesterol content.

Cholesterol also partitions into specialized regions of the membrane called lipid rafts microdomains enriched in cholesterol and sphingolipids that are more densely packed and less fluid than the surrounding bilayer. Lipid rafts serve as organizational platforms for particular membrane proteins, especially those involved in signal transduction. Many signaling receptors, ion channels, and enzymes preferentially associate with lipid rafts, and the disruption of raft formation impairs cellular signaling.

Beyond its structural role in membranes, cholesterol is the precursor to a remarkable array of biologically active molecules. In the adrenal cortex, cholesterol is converted to the glucocorticoids (cortisol) and mineralocorticoids (aldosterone) that regulate metabolism and blood pressure. In the gonads, it is converted to the sex hormones testosterone and estradiol. In the liver, it is converted to bile acids the detergent-like molecules that emulsify dietary fat in the small intestine. In the skin, it is converted by ultraviolet light to cholecalciferol, the precursor to vitamin D.

3.5 Lipid Signaling: When Fat Becomes a Messenger

The idea that fat molecules serve not only as structural and storage materials but also as precise molecular signals capable of conveying specific biological messages from one cell to another or from one part of a cell to another — is one of the most exciting developments in modern biology.

Eicosanoids are a family of lipid signaling molecules derived from 20-carbon polyunsaturated fatty acids, particularly arachidonic acid. The word "eicosanoid" comes from the Greek "eikosi," meaning twenty. Eicosanoids include prostaglandins, thromboxanes, leukotrienes, and lipoxins each with distinct biological activities and produced by different cell types in response to different stimuli.

Prostaglandins are among the most potent and locally acting of all biological signaling molecules. They are produced by virtually every cell type and act primarily on neighboring cells (paracrine signaling) or on the cell that produced them (autocrine signaling). Different prostaglandins can cause constriction or dilation of blood vessels, stimulate or inhibit platelet aggregation, promote or reduce inflammation, induce smooth muscle contraction (prostaglandins are responsible for the uterine contractions of labor), and modulate pain sensitivity by sensitizing nociceptors (pain receptors) to stimulation.

Aspirin, one of the world's most widely used drugs, works by irreversibly inhibiting the enzyme cyclooxygenase (COX), which catalyzes the first committed step in prostaglandin synthesis. By blocking prostaglandin production, aspirin reduces fever, inflammation, and pain and reduces the risk of blood clot formation by inhibiting thromboxane A2, a prostaglandin that promotes platelet aggregation. The discovery of COX-2-specific inhibitors (the so-called "COX-2 inhibitors" like celecoxib) provided anti-inflammatory drugs with fewer gastrointestinal side effects than traditional aspirin-like drugs.

Phosphatidylinositol-based signaling represents another major lipid signaling pathway. When certain cell surface receptors are activated, they trigger the hydrolysis of phosphatidylinositol 4,5-bisphosphate (PIP2) in the cell membrane to produce two second messengers: diacylglycerol (DAG), which remains in the membrane and activates protein kinase C, and inositol 1,4,5-trisphosphate (IP3), which diffuses through the cytoplasm to trigger calcium release from the endoplasmic reticulum. This calcium signal, amplified and shaped by various cellular mechanisms, can activate enzymes, trigger secretion, initiate muscle contraction, or alter gene expression.

Sphingolipid metabolism also produces important signaling molecules. Ceramide a sphingolipid backbone without a head group is a potent inducer of apoptosis (programmed cell death). Sphingosine-1-phosphate (S1P) promotes cell survival and stimulates lymphocyte trafficking. The balance between ceramide and S1P sometimes called the sphingolipid rheostat is an important determinant of cell fate: survival versus death.

Chapter Summary

Lipids are unified not by a common covalent structure but by hydrophobicity their tendency to be insoluble in water and soluble in non-polar solvents. This property arises from their long hydrocarbon chains and/or fused ring systems, which lack the polar groups necessary for favorable interactions with water.

Fatty acids carboxylic acids with long hydrocarbon tails are the building blocks of most lipid classes. Their saturation state (the presence or absence of double bonds) determines their physical state and biological properties. Triglycerides, formed from glycerol and three fatty acids, are the primary energy storage form in animals compact, anhydrous, and energy-dense.

Phospholipids, with their amphipathic structure (polar head, non-polar tails), spontaneously form the lipid bilayers of cell membranes. Cholesterol regulates membrane fluidity and serves as the precursor to steroid hormones, bile acids, and vitamin D. Lipid signaling molecules eicosanoids, inositol phosphates, and sphingolipids mediate inflammation, pain, calcium signaling, and cell survival decisions.

Having explored carbohydrates and lipids, we now turn to perhaps the most versatile and structurally elaborate of all biomolecule classes: proteins. These molecular workhorses carry out virtually every active function of the cell, from catalyzing chemical reactions to transmitting signals to building the cytoskeleton. Their story begins with amino acids.

CHAPTER 4

Proteins: The Molecular Workhorses of the Cell

Amino Acids, Peptide Bonds, and Protein Architecture

Consider for a moment the staggering breadth of what proteins do. They catalyze the chemical reactions of metabolism, at rates millions of times faster than those reactions would proceed without them. They form the structural scaffolding of cells and tissues the collagen of skin, the actin of muscle, the tubulin of the cytoskeleton. They transport oxygen through the blood (hemoglobin), carry lipids between tissues (albumin), and shuttle electrons along the mitochondrial membrane (cytochrome c). They receive signals from the environment, transmit those signals inside the cell, and execute the appropriate responses. They defend the body against pathogens (antibodies). They regulate which genes are turned on or off (transcription factors). They build new proteins (ribosomes are largely protein). They even break down old proteins (proteases).

There is no overstatement possible in characterizing the importance of proteins. Every metabolic transformation, every cellular response, every act of development, every immune defense all of it is carried out by proteins. And underlying this extraordinary functional diversity is a structural principle of astonishing simplicity: proteins are linear polymers of amino acids, folded into precise three-dimensional shapes. The sequence of amino acids in a protein encoded in DNA ultimately determines the protein's shape, and its shape determines its function. This is the central insight of structural biology, and it is one of the most profound ideas in all of science.

4.1 The Amino Acid Alphabet: Twenty Letters, Infinite Words

Amino acids are the monomers of proteins. There are 20 standard amino acids used in biological protein synthesis (a few rare additional amino acids, like selenocysteine and pyrrolysine, are incorporated by specialized mechanisms in some organisms). Every protein in every living cell from the simplest bacterium to the most complex mammal is built from combinations of these same 20 amino acids.

All 20 standard amino acids share a common structural core. At the center is a carbon atom called the alpha-carbon (Cα). Attached to this carbon are four groups: an amino group ($-NH_2$), a carboxyl group (–COOH), a hydrogen atom, and a side chain called the R group. It is the R group that differs between amino acids and that gives each amino acid its distinct chemical character. The amino group and carboxyl group are what allow amino acids to form peptide bonds and join into chains. The R group is what makes each amino acid unique.

The 20 amino acids can be grouped by the chemical properties of their R groups a classification that is enormously helpful for understanding protein structure and function. The first major division is between non-polar (hydrophobic) and polar amino acids.

Non-polar amino acids have R groups that are predominantly hydrocarbon chains or rings of carbon and hydrogen with no polar atoms. These include glycine (the smallest, with just a hydrogen as its R group), alanine, valine, leucine, isoleucine, proline, phenylalanine, tryptophan, and methionine. Non-polar amino acids are the "oil-loving" members of the protein family they tend to cluster in the interior of folded proteins, away from the aqueous environment, driven by the same hydrophobic effect that causes oil to separate from water.

Polar uncharged amino acids have R groups with polar functional groups (hydroxyl, thiol, amide) but are not charged at physiological pH. These include serine, threonine, cysteine, tyrosine, asparagine, and glutamine. Their polar groups can form hydrogen bonds with water and with other polar groups in the protein, making them suitable for protein surfaces and active sites.

Charged amino acids bear either a positive charge (basic amino acids: lysine, arginine, and histidine) or a negative charge (acidic amino acids: aspartate and glutamate) at physiological pH. These amino acids are strongly hydrophilic and are typically found on the protein's surface, where they can interact with the aqueous environment. They are also critical players in enzyme active sites, where their charges can facilitate the binding of substrates or the catalytic chemistry of reactions.

The properties of the 20 amino acids are not merely chemical curiosities they are the functional vocabulary from which protein structures are built. Every time a protein folds, it does so because the specific amino acid sequence, interacting with itself and with water, spontaneously adopts the thermodynamically most stable three-dimensional arrangement. Understanding the properties of each amino acid is the first step toward understanding how and why proteins fold the way they do.

4.2 The Peptide Bond: Chemistry's Covalent Protein Link

Amino acids are linked into proteins by peptide bonds covalent bonds formed between the carboxyl group of one amino acid and the amino group of the next, with the release of a water molecule in a condensation reaction. This reaction is thermodynamically unfavorable in isolation (it requires energy input) and is driven in cells by the ribosome, which couple's peptide bond formation to the hydrolysis of high-energy GTP molecules.

The resulting bond the peptide bond has a remarkable and unexpected property: it has partial double-bond character. The nitrogen atom of the peptide bond donates electron density to the carbonyl carbon, creating a resonance structure in which the C–N bond is about 40% double bond in character. This prevents free rotation around the C–N bond unlike ordinary single bonds, which can rotate freely and forces the six atoms of the peptide bond (Cα, C, O, N, H, and the next Cα) to be coplanar.

This planarity of the peptide bond has profound consequences for protein structure. It means that the peptide backbone of a protein is not a completely flexible chain rotation is restricted to two specific bonds in each amino acid residue: the bond between the alpha-carbon and the nitrogen (the ϕ, or phi, bond) and the bond between the alpha-carbon and the carbonyl carbon (the ψ, or psi, bond). The allowed combinations of ϕ and ψ angles plotted on a diagram called the Ramachandran plot define the backbone conformations that are sterically accessible to a polypeptide chain, and these accessible conformations correspond to the regular secondary structures of proteins: alpha helices and beta sheets.

The formation of a peptide bond creates a polypeptide chain with a defined directionality: one end bears a free amino group (the N-terminus or amino terminus) and the other bears a free carboxyl group (the C-terminus or carboxyl terminus). By convention, protein sequences are always written from N-terminus to C-terminus, left to right. This directionality analogous to the 5' to 3' directionality of nucleic acids is biologically meaningful: ribosomes synthesize proteins exclusively in the N-to-C direction, and the information encoded in mRNA is read in the 5'-to-3' direction.

4.3 Secondary Structure: The Regular Folds of the Protein Backbone

Protein secondary structure refers to the locally regular patterns of backbone folding that arise from hydrogen bonding between backbone NH and C=O groups. These patterns are consistent and predictable they recur in the same forms in proteins of vastly different amino acid sequences and functions because they represent the geometrically optimal ways for the protein backbone to form intramolecular hydrogen bonds.

The alpha helix is the most visually iconic element of protein secondary structure. In an alpha helix, the polypeptide backbone winds into a right-handed spiral, with 3.6 amino acid residues per turn and a rise of 1.5 Å per residue (giving a pitch of 5.4 Å per turn). The helix is stabilized by hydrogen bonds between the carbonyl oxygen of residue n and the amide nitrogen of residue n+4 that is, every backbone C=O is hydrogen-bonded to the backbone N–H that is four residues ahead of it in the chain. The R groups of the amino acids project outward from the helical backbone, away from the axis of the helix.

Alpha helices are remarkably stable structures, and they are found in an enormous variety of proteins. Transmembrane helices segments of 20–25 hydrophobic amino acids that span the lipid bilayer are alpha helices that anchor membrane proteins in the membrane. The muscle proteins myosin and tropomyosin form extended alpha-helical coiled-coil structures. Many transcription factors use alpha helices to bind specific DNA sequences. The structural protein keratin making up hair, nails, and the outer layer of skin is built almost entirely from coiled-coil alpha helices.

The beta sheet is the other major element of protein secondary structure. In a beta sheet, two or more segments of the polypeptide backbone (called beta strands) lie adjacent to each other and form hydrogen bonds between their backbone groups. Unlike the alpha helix, which involves hydrogen bonding within a single continuous stretch of chain, the beta sheet involves hydrogen bonding between strands that may be far apart in the protein sequence.

Beta strands can be arranged in two ways: parallel (running in the same N-to-C direction) or antiparallel (running in opposite directions). Antiparallel beta sheets are somewhat more stable because the hydrogen bonds are more linear. Both parallel and antiparallel beta sheets are widely found in proteins. The immunoglobulin fold the structural scaffold of antibodies is built around a characteristic antiparallel beta-sheet sandwich. The serine proteases (enzymes that cut proteins, including many digestive enzymes and blood clotting factors) have a barrel-like structure formed by a set of beta strands curled into a cylinder.

Between regions of alpha helix and beta sheet, protein chains often contain short, irregular segments called loops or turns. These provide the architectural connections between the regular secondary structure elements. Far from being unimportant spacers, loops are often the most functionally critical parts of a protein they form the binding sites for substrates and cofactors, the recognition surfaces for other proteins, and the catalytic residues of enzyme active sites.

4.4 Tertiary and Quaternary Structure: The Full Three-Dimensional Architecture

Secondary structure describes the local folding of the protein backbone. Tertiary structure describes the global three-dimensional arrangement of all the atoms in a single polypeptide chain the way the secondary structure elements are packed and arranged relative to each other. It is the tertiary structure that gives a protein its specific shape, and therefore its specific function.

The forces that stabilize tertiary structure are the same forces that govern molecular interactions throughout all of chemistry, operating in the context of the polypeptide chain and the aqueous environment.

The hydrophobic effect is the dominant force in protein folding. As a protein folds, non-polar amino acid side chains are driven together to form a compact hydrophobic core, away from the surrounding water. This burial of hydrophobic surfaces is thermodynamically favorable (it increases the entropy of the surrounding water molecules that would otherwise be organized around non-polar surfaces). The hydrophobic core of a folded protein is so densely packed that it resembles the interior of a crystal rather than a liquid a remarkable level of molecular complementarity achieved without template or mold.

Hydrogen bonds between polar R groups, and between R groups and backbone atoms, add specificity to the folded structure. Although individual hydrogen bonds are weak (about 1-3 kcal/mol), a protein may contain hundreds of them, and their cumulative contribution to stability is substantial.

Ionic interactions between oppositely charged R groups called salt bridges can also stabilize protein structure, particularly at the protein's surface. Disulfide bonds covalent bonds between the sulfhydryl groups of cysteine residues are the most stable structural elements in extracellular proteins, where they provide resistance to the reducing and unfolding conditions of the extracellular environment. Insulin, immunoglobulins, and many secreted enzymes rely on disulfide bonds for their stability.

Van der Waals forces the weak, short-range attractive forces between adjacent atoms due to transient fluctuations in electron distribution are individually tiny but collectively important. They are the forces responsible for the exquisite fit between different surfaces in the protein interior.

Quaternary structure refers to the association of two or more polypeptide chains (subunits) into a single functional protein complex. Many biologically important proteins are multimeric they consist of multiple polypeptide chains held together by the same non-covalent forces that stabilize tertiary structure.

Hemoglobin, the oxygen-carrying protein of red blood cells, is a classic example. It consists of four subunits: two alpha chains and two beta chains, each of which carries one heme group (an iron-containing prosthetic group that binds oxygen). The quaternary structure of hemoglobin is not merely a structural elaboration it enables a property called cooperativity, in which the binding of oxygen to one subunit changes the affinity of the other subunits for oxygen. This cooperative binding gives hemoglobin its sigmoidal oxygen-binding curve, which makes it an efficient oxygen carrier in the lungs and an efficient oxygen deliverer to the tissues.

4.5 Protein Folding and Misfolding: When Things Go Wrong

The folding of a newly synthesized polypeptide chain into its correct three-dimensional structure is one of the most remarkable and most biologically risky processes in the cell. A chain of several hundred amino acids has an astronomical number of possible conformations, yet it reaches its correct folded structure in milliseconds to seconds. How does it navigate this immense conformational space so rapidly?

Theoretical considerations first raised by Cyrus Levinthal in the 1960s (now known as the Levinthal paradox) showed that if a protein sampled all possible conformations randomly before settling on the correct one, the process would take longer than the age of the universe. The actual speed of protein folding often completed in microseconds to seconds implies that folding is not random but directed: it follows a pathway guided by local interactions that progressively constrain the chain's conformation toward the native structure.

The current model of protein folding is based on the concept of an energy landscape a multidimensional surface representing the energy of the protein as a function of its conformation. Folding proceeds by the protein "rolling downhill" on this landscape toward the lowest-energy conformation (the native state). The landscape is not smooth but funnel-shaped there are many high-energy conformations at the top (unfolded states) and fewer, lower-energy conformations closer to the native state. This funnel-shaped landscape guides folding efficiently without requiring systematic sampling of all possible conformations.

In the crowded interior of a cell, protein folding is assisted by specialized proteins called molecular chaperones. Chaperones do not determine the final structure of a protein (that is determined by the amino acid sequence) but rather prevent premature or incorrect folding by binding to exposed hydrophobic regions of nascent or partially folded chains. The major chaperone families the Hsp70 family, the chaperonins (like GroEL in bacteria and TRiC in eukaryotes), and the Hsp90 family work together to ensure that proteins achieve their correct folded states.

When proteins misfold, the consequences can be catastrophic. Misfolded proteins frequently expose hydrophobic regions that cause them to aggregate with other misfolded proteins, forming insoluble clumps called amyloid fibrils. These fibrillar aggregates are associated with a growing list of devastating human diseases including Alzheimer's disease (aggregation of amyloid-beta and tau), Parkinson's disease (aggregation of alpha-synuclein), Huntington's disease (aggregation of huntingtin), type 2 diabetes (aggregation of islet amyloid polypeptide), and the transmissible spongiform encephalopathies or prion diseases (aggregation of prion protein). Understanding how and why proteins misfold is one of the most urgently important problems in biomolecular science today.

Chapter Summary

Proteins are the molecular workhorses of the cell performing virtually every active biological function from catalysis to structural support, from signaling to immune defense. Their remarkable functional diversity flows from a structural principle of elegant simplicity: linear polymers of amino acids, folded into precise three-dimensional shapes.

The 20 standard amino acids, each with a distinct R group, constitute the chemical alphabet of proteins. Their properties hydrophobic, polar, acidic, basic determine the folding of polypeptide chains through the hydrophobic effect, hydrogen bonding, ionic interactions, van der Waals forces, and disulfide bonds.

Protein structure is organized into four levels: primary (amino acid sequence), secondary (alpha helices and beta sheets stabilized by backbone hydrogen bonds), tertiary (overall three-dimensional fold), and quaternary (association of multiple subunits). Protein folding follows a funnel-shaped energy landscape, guided by local interactions and assisted by molecular chaperones. Misfolding leads to aggregation and the amyloid fibrils associated with neurodegenerative diseases.

CHAPTER 5

Enzymes: Nature's Catalysts

Kinetics, Mechanisms, and Regulation of Enzymatic Activity

In a laboratory flask at room temperature, sucrose ordinary table sugar will sit in aqueous solution essentially unchanged for years. The reaction of sucrose hydrolysis (its breakdown into glucose and fructose) is thermodynamically favorable it releases energy but it is so incredibly slow without a catalyst that no spontaneous breakdown is measurable on any practical timescale. Add a small amount of the enzyme sucrase (also called invertase), however, and the sucrose is completely hydrolyzed in seconds.

This transformation from geological timescale to seconds illustrates the extraordinary catalytic power of enzymes. These biological catalysts accelerate chemical reactions by factors ranging from one million to one billion billion (10^{18}) times over the uncatalyzed rate. They do so with exquisite specificity each enzyme catalyzes essentially just one reaction, or one type of reaction, among the many thousands of chemical reactions that occur simultaneously in a cell. And they do so under mild conditions at body temperature, near-neutral pH, in aqueous solution without the high temperatures, extreme pH values, or exotic organic solvents that industrial chemical processes often require.

Enzymes are proteins (with a small number of exceptions certain RNA molecules, called ribozymes, also have catalytic activity, as discussed in Chapter 6). Their catalytic activity depends entirely on their three-dimensional structure on the precise geometric and chemical arrangement of their active site. Denature an enzyme (unfold it with heat or detergent), and its catalytic activity is destroyed, because the active site is disrupted. Restore the native structure (if possible), and catalytic activity returns.

This chapter explores the principles of enzymatic catalysis: how enzymes bind their substrates, how they lower activation energy, what kinetic laws govern their activity, and how their activity is regulated to meet the metabolic needs of the cell.

5.1 The Active Site: Where Chemistry Happens

An enzyme is typically a large globular protein of many hundreds of amino acid residues, yet its catalytic activity is localized to a small region of its three-dimensional structure called the active site. The active site is a pocket or cleft on the enzyme's surface formed by the folding of the polypeptide chain whose shape and chemical properties are precisely complementary to the substrate (the molecule being transformed) and to the transition state of the reaction.

The active site contains two functionally distinct types of residues. Binding residues amino acids that form non-covalent interactions (hydrogen bonds, ionic interactions, hydrophobic contacts, van der Waals forces) with the substrate hold the substrate in the correct orientation and position for catalysis. Catalytic residues a smaller set of amino acids at the core of the active site are directly involved in the chemical transformation: they may donate or accept protons, form covalent intermediates with the substrate, stabilize charged transition states, or activate water molecules for nucleophilic attack.

The complementarity between the enzyme's active site and its substrate is not static but dynamic. In the earliest model of enzyme-substrate interaction the "lock and key" model proposed by Emil Fischer in 1894 the enzyme was thought of as a rigid lock into which the substrate key fits perfectly. This model explained specificity but failed to account for several observations. The modern "induced fit" model, proposed by Daniel Koshland in 1958, recognizes that both the enzyme and the substrate undergo conformational changes when they interact. The binding of the substrate induces a change in the shape of the active site that achieves an even more perfect fit optimizing the geometric and chemical complementarity between enzyme and substrate.

The catalytic power of enzymes arises from their ability to stabilize the transition state the highest-energy, most unstable arrangement of atoms along the reaction pathway. By binding the transition state more tightly than either the substrate or the products, the enzyme effectively lowers the activation energy of the reaction. The substrate enters the active site, the enzyme reshapes itself around the substrate, and the active site environment through strategic placement of charged, polar, and hydrogen-bonding groups creates a microenvironment that specifically stabilizes the transition state. The result is a reaction pathway that circumvents the high-energy barrier of the uncatalyzed reaction.

5.2 Michaelis-Menten Kinetics: The Mathematics of Enzymatic Speed

In 1913, Leonor Michaelis and Maud Menten published a mathematical treatment of enzyme kinetics that remains, over a century later, the foundation of quantitative enzymology. Their model describes how the rate of an enzyme-catalyzed reaction depends on the concentration of substrate, and it captures the essential behavior of most enzymes with just two parameters: the Michaelis constant (Km) and the maximum velocity (Vmax).

The Michaelis-Menten model begins with a simple mechanistic proposal: an enzyme (E) binds reversibly to its substrate (S) to form an enzyme-substrate complex (ES), which then breaks down to release the product (P) and regenerate the free enzyme. The rate of the overall reaction depends on how much ES complex is present which in turn depends on substrate concentration.

At very low substrate concentrations, only a small fraction of the enzyme molecules is occupied with substrate at any given time. The reaction rate is proportional to substrate concentration doubling the substrate doubles the rate. At very high substrate concentrations, essentially all the enzyme molecules are occupied with substrate all the time the enzyme is saturated. Adding more substrate cannot increase the rate, because there is no free enzyme available to bind it. The reaction rate reaches a ceiling called Vmax (maximum velocity).

The Km (Michaelis constant) is the substrate concentration at which the reaction rate is exactly half of Vmax. It is a useful indicator of the affinity of an enzyme for its substrate: a low Km means the enzyme reaches half-maximum velocity at a low substrate concentration implying high affinity. A high Km means the enzyme needs a high substrate concentration to reach half-maximum rate implying lower affinity.

The Michaelis-Menten equation elegantly summarizes all of this: $V = (Vmax \times [S]) / (Km + [S])$. This hyperbolic relationship between substrate concentration and reaction rate when plotted gives the characteristic saturation curve of enzymology: a rapid rise at low substrate concentrations that gradually levels off at high concentrations as the enzyme approaches saturation.

Another important enzyme parameter is the turnover number, or kcat the number of substrate molecules converted to product per enzyme molecule per second when the enzyme is fully saturated. Carbonic anhydrase, the enzyme that converts CO_2 to bicarbonate in red blood cells, has a kcat of about 600,000 per second it processes 600,000 molecules of CO_2 every second per enzyme molecule, making it one of the fastest enzymes known. By contrast, lysozyme, which cleaves bacterial cell walls, has a kcat of about 0.5 per second.

The ratio kcat/Km called the specificity constant is arguably the most useful single measure of enzyme efficiency. It reflects both how tightly an enzyme binds its substrate (Km) and how quickly it processes it (kcat). The theoretical upper limit of kcat/Km is set by the diffusion limit the rate at which substrate molecules randomly collide with enzyme molecules in solution, approximately 10^8–10^9 $M^{-1}s^{-1}$. Enzymes that have reached this limit called "catalytically perfect" enzymes include triose phosphate isomerase, acetylcholinesterase, and catalase.

5.3 Enzyme Inhibition: Slowing the Molecular Machine

The ability to inhibit specific enzymes is one of the most powerful tools in pharmacology and biochemistry. Many drugs, toxins, and natural regulatory molecules work by inhibiting enzymes reducing their catalytic activity by interfering with substrate binding or catalytic mechanism. Understanding the types of enzyme inhibition not only illuminates how these substances work but provides a framework for rational drug design.

Competitive inhibitors are molecules that resemble the substrate and compete with it for binding to the active site. When a competitive inhibitor is bound, the substrate cannot bind, and vice versa they are mutually exclusive. Because the inhibitor must compete with the substrate, the effect of a competitive inhibitor can be overcome by increasing the substrate concentration. In the language of Michaelis-Menten kinetics, competitive inhibition increases the apparent Km (because more substrate is needed to displace the inhibitor) but does not affect Vmax (because at infinitely high substrate concentration, the substrate wins the competition completely).

Statins the most widely prescribed class of drugs in the world, used to lower cholesterol are competitive inhibitors of HMG-CoA reductase, the rate-limiting enzyme in the cholesterol biosynthesis pathway. They closely resemble the enzyme's natural substrate, HMG-CoA, and bind to the active site with higher affinity than the substrate itself, thereby reducing cholesterol synthesis.

Non-competitive inhibitors bind to a site on the enzyme that is separate from the active site called the allosteric site and reduce enzyme activity by changing the enzyme's conformation in a way that reduces catalytic efficiency. Because the non-competitive inhibitor does not compete with the substrate for the active site, adding more substrate does not overcome the inhibition. In Michaelis-Menten terms, non-competitive inhibition reduces Vmax without changing Km.

Uncompetitive inhibitors bind exclusively to the enzyme-substrate complex (ES), not to the free enzyme. They reduce both Km and Vmax by the same factor a distinctive kinetic signature that can be identified on a Lineweaver-Burk plot (a double-reciprocal transformation of the Michaelis-Menten equation used for graphical analysis).

Irreversible inhibitors form covalent bonds with amino acid residues in the active site, permanently inactivating the enzyme. Organophosphate nerve agents (like sarin and VX) and certain pesticides work by irreversibly inhibiting acetylcholinesterase, the enzyme that terminates nerve signals by breaking down the neurotransmitter acetylcholine. When acetylcholinesterase is inhibited, acetylcholine accumulates at nerve synapses, causing continuous nerve firing and ultimately fatal muscle paralysis and convulsions.

Aspirin, as mentioned in Chapter 3, irreversibly inhibits cyclooxygenase (COX) enzymes through acetylation of a serine residue in the active site. This irreversible inhibition is why aspirin's antiplatelet effects last for the lifetime of the platelet (about 10 days) platelets cannot synthesize new COX because they have no nuclei, so once their COX is acetylated, it is permanently inactivated.

5.4 Allosteric Regulation: The Enzyme's Molecular Dimmer Switch

Many enzymes particularly those that control key branch points or committed steps in metabolic pathways are not simply switched on or off but are fine-tuned: their activity is adjusted up or down in response to signals from the cellular environment. The primary mechanism of this fine-tuning is allosteric regulation.

Allosteric enzymes have two types of binding sites: the active site where substrate binds and the allosteric site (or sites) where regulatory molecules bind. The binding of a regulatory molecule to the allosteric site induces a conformational change in the enzyme a change in shape that alters the properties of the active site. If this conformational change increases catalytic activity, the regulatory molecule is an allosteric activator. If it decreases activity, it is an allosteric inhibitor.

Allosteric enzymes typically display sigmoidal (S-shaped) rather than hyperbolic kinetics their activity increases steeply over a narrow range of substrate concentrations. This sigmoidal behavior arises from cooperativity: the binding of one substrate molecule changes the affinity of the enzyme for subsequent substrate molecules, making the enzyme more sensitive to changes in substrate concentration than a simple Michaelis-Menten enzyme would be.

Feedback inhibition is among the most elegant forms of metabolic regulation. In a biosynthetic pathway a series of enzyme-catalyzed steps that converts a starting material into a final product the end product often serves as an allosteric inhibitor of the first enzyme in the pathway. This creates an automatic self-regulating circuit: when the end product accumulates (indicating that production is exceeding demand), it feeds back to inhibit the first enzyme and slow down the entire pathway. When the end product is consumed (indicating that demand exceeds production), inhibition is relieved, and the pathway speeds up.

The regulation of AT Case (aspartate transcarboxylase) by CTP (cytidine triphosphate) is the classic example. AT Case catalyzes the first committed step of pyrimidine nucleotide biosynthesis. When CTP levels are high, CTP binds to the allosteric site of AT Case and inhibits its activity, slowing pyrimidine synthesis. When CTP levels fall, inhibition is relieved, and pyrimidine synthesis accelerates. This simple feedback loop keeps pyrimidine nucleotide production tightly coupled to cellular demand.

5.5 Coenzymes, Cofactors, and Vitamins: The Essential Partners of Enzymes

Many enzymes cannot function on their own they require additional non-protein chemical components called cofactors to carry out their catalytic function. This requirement for cofactors is one of the reasons why certain minerals and vitamins are essential for life: they serve as enzyme cofactors, and without them, critical metabolic reactions cannot proceed.

Cofactors can be either inorganic ions or organic molecules. Inorganic ion cofactors include metal ions like zinc (Zn^{2+}), magnesium (Mg^{2+}), iron (Fe^{2+}/Fe^{3+}), copper (Cu^{2+}), manganese (Mn^{2+}), and cobalt (Co^{2+}). Metal ions can participate directly in catalytic reactions (facilitating electron transfer, activating water molecules, or stabilizing charged intermediates) or can help maintain the active site structure.

Organic cofactors are called coenzymes. Unlike the enzyme protein itself, coenzymes are changed by the reaction and must be regenerated (either by a separate reaction or as part of the overall metabolic pathway). The most important coenzymes in biology include NAD+ (nicotinamide adenine dinucleotide), FAD (flavin adenine dinucleotide), coenzyme A (CoA), tetrahydrofolate (THF), and pyridoxal phosphate (PLP).

Many coenzymes are derived from vitamins small organic molecules that humans (and many other animals) cannot synthesize themselves and must obtain from their diet. This is why the word "vitamin" (from "vital amine" though not all vitamins are amines) refers to essential dietary factors: they are the precursors to coenzymes that are indispensable for metabolic function.

NAD+ is derived from niacin (vitamin B3). It functions as a carrier of electrons (hydride ions, H^-) in oxidation-reduction reactions of metabolism accepting electrons from metabolites being oxidized and carrying them to the electron transport chain, where they are used to drive ATP synthesis. Severe niacin deficiency causes pellagra, a disease characterized by skin rashes, diarrhea, dementia, and death a consequence of impaired NAD+ availability and the resulting failure of metabolic energy production.

Coenzyme A, derived from pantothenic acid (vitamin B5), is the universal carrier of acetyl groups in metabolism. Acetyl-CoA is the entry molecule for the citric acid cycle and the starting material for fatty acid and steroid synthesis. The "coenzyme A" portion does the carrying it forms a thioester bond with acetyl groups while pantothenic acid contributes to its structure.

Chapter Summary

Enzymes are biological catalysts of extraordinary power and specificity. They accelerate reactions by lowering activation energy primarily by stabilizing the transition state of the reaction through the precise geometric and chemical environment of their active sites. The induced-fit model describes how both enzyme and substrate change shape upon binding, achieving optimal complementarity.

Michaelis-Menten kinetics provides the quantitative framework for analyzing enzyme behavior. The parameters Km (substrate affinity indicator) and Vmax (maximum rate at saturating substrate), along with kcat (turnover number) and the specificity constant kcat/Km, characterize enzyme performance and guide drug design.

Enzyme inhibitors competitive, non-competitive, uncompetitive, and irreversible are among the most important classes of pharmacological agents. Allosteric regulation allows enzymes to serve as metabolic sensors and rheostats, adjusting pathway flux in response to the cell's current needs. Cofactors and coenzymes many derived from vitamins are the essential partners of enzymes, providing chemical functionality that protein side chains alone cannot deliver.

Having explored the protein catalyst, we now turn to the molecules that store and transmit the instructions for making every protein in every cell: the nucleic acids, DNA and RNA.

CHAPTER 6

Nucleic Acids: Blueprints of Biological Information

The Structure and Function of DNA and RNA

In 1944, Oswald Avery, Colin MacLeod, and Maclyn McCarty published one of the most important and initially most disbelieved papers in the history of biology. They showed that the "transforming principle" that could change harmless bacteria into lethal ones was not protein (as most scientists at the time assumed) but deoxyribonucleic acid: DNA. The scientific community was skeptical. Proteins, with their 20 different amino acids and virtually unlimited structural diversity, seemed far better candidates for the repository of genetic information than DNA, with its apparently simple composition of just four nucleotide bases. Surely, the biological library of hereditary information could not be written in

an alphabet of only four letters.

They were wrong gloriously, productively wrong. An alphabet of four letters, arranged in sequences of billions, can store information of unimaginable richness. The human genome contains approximately 3.2 billion base pairs of DNAS, encoding the instructions for building and operating every cell, tissue, and organ of the human body. If you printed out the human genome at one letter per millimeter the resulting scroll would stretch from London to Tokyo and back, five times over.

Nucleic acids DNA and RNA are the information molecules of life. They store genetic information, transmit it between generations, and direct its expression into the proteins that carry out all biological functions. This chapter explores the chemical structure of nucleic acids, the double helical architecture of DNA, the functional diversity of RNA molecules, and the way that DNA is packaged into chromosomes.

6.1 Nucleotides: The Four-Letter Alphabet of Life

Nucleic acids are polymers of nucleotides the monomeric building blocks of both DNA and RNA. A nucleotide consists of three components covalently linked together: a nitrogenous base, a five-carbon (pentose) sugar, and one or more phosphate groups.

The nitrogenous bases are flat, aromatic ring structures containing nitrogen atoms. They are divided into two chemical families: purines (with a fused double-ring structure) and pyrimidines (with a single ring). In DNA, the purines are adenine (A) and guanine (G), and the pyrimidines are cytosine (C) and thymine (T). In RNA, thymine is replaced by uracil (U) a structurally similar pyrimidine that lacks the methyl group found on thymine's ring. The identity of the base is what carries the genetic information the sequence of bases along a nucleic acid chain is the sequence of the genetic code.

The sugar component of a DNA nucleotide is 2'-deoxyribose a ribose sugar lacking the hydroxyl group at the 2' carbon position. RNA contains ribose the same sugar with the 2' hydroxyl intact. This single chemical difference one oxygen atom has profound structural and functional consequences. The 2'-OH, of RNA makes it more chemically reactive (and therefore less chemically stable) than DNA. RNA can be cleaved by hydrolysis under mildly basic conditions that leave DNA intact, because the 2'-OH can participate in a cyclization reaction that attacks the adjacent phosphodiester bond. This greater reactivity of RNA relative to DNA is one reason why DNA evolved as the long-term repository of genetic information it is simply more stable.

Nucleotides are linked into chains by phosphodiester bonds bonds in which a phosphate group bridges the 3'-oxygen of one sugar and the 5'-oxygen of the next. The result is an unbranched polymer with a repeating phosphate-sugar backbone and a sequence of bases projecting from this backbone. The backbone carries a strong negative charge two of the four oxygen atoms on each phosphate group are ionized at physiological pH making nucleic acids among the most strongly negatively charged biological molecules.

The chain has directionality: one end has a free 5'-phosphate group (the 5' end) and the other has a free 3'-hydroxyl group (the 3' end). By convention, nucleotide sequences are written 5' to 3', from left to right. This 5'-to-3' directionality is biologically fundamental DNA is replicated in the 5'-to-3' direction, RNA is synthesized in the 5'-to-3' direction, and ribosomes translate mRNA in the 5'-to-3' direction.

6.2 The DNA Double Helix: Nature's Master Archive

The discovery of the structure of DNA in 1953 by Watson and Crick informed by the X-ray crystallographic work of Rosalind Franklin and Raymond Gosling is one of the great intellectual achievements of the twentieth century. The publication of their famous paper in Nature ran to less than a single page, yet it contained a sentence of extraordinary understatement: "It has not escaped our notice that the specific pairing we have postulated immediately suggests a possible copying mechanism for the genetic material."

The double helix consists of two antiparallel DNA strands (running in opposite 5'-to-3' directions) wound around a common central axis in a right-handed helix. The sugar-phosphate backbones are on the outside of the helix, exposed to the aqueous environment. The bases project inward, stacking on top of each other in the center of the helix and pairing specifically with bases on the opposite strand.

Base pairing is governed by strict complementarity: adenine pairs with thymine (A–T), forming two hydrogen bonds, and guanine pairs with cytosine (G–C), forming three hydrogen bonds. This complementary base pairing known as Watson-Crick base pairing is the key to virtually everything that DNA does. It allows DNA to be accurately copied (because each strand serves as a template for the synthesis of a new complementary strand). It allows genetic information to be read (because the sequence of one strand determines the sequence of its complement). And it allows the double helix to be stable despite being held together only by non-covalent interactions.

The bases in the double helix are stacked on top of each other with an inter-base spacing of 3.4 Å. This stacking is stabilized by pi-pi interactions the attraction between the flat aromatic ring systems of adjacent bases. Base stacking is actually a larger contributor to the stability of the double helix than Watson-Crick hydrogen bonding unwinding the two strands of a double helix requires disrupting both hydrogen bonds and stacking interactions.

The canonical form of the DNA double helix described by Watson and Crick is called B-DNA. It has 10.5 base pairs per turn of the helix, a helical pitch of 34 Å, and distinct major and minor grooves widened and narrowed regions of the helix where the bases are accessible from the outside. The major groove is wider and deeper, and it is the region where most DNA-binding proteins (transcription factors, restriction enzymes, etc.) make contact with specific base sequences.

Alternative DNA conformations A-DNA (a wider, shorter helix that forms in dehydrated conditions), Z-DNA (a left-handed helix that forms in sequences of alternating purines and pyrimidines) also exist and may play roles in gene regulation, but B-DNA is the predominant form in cells under physiological conditions.

6.3 The RNA Universe: One Polymer, Many Faces

For decades after the discovery of the double helix, RNA was thought of as a relatively humble molecule a passive messenger carrying information from DNA to the protein synthesis machinery, plus the structural and functional RNA molecules of the ribosome. The RNA world has turned out to be vastly richer and more complex than this simple picture suggested.

Messenger RNA (mRNA) is the information-carrying RNA the transcript of a gene that is translated by the ribosome into a protein sequence. In eukaryotes, mRNA is initially synthesized as a long precursor (pre-mRNA) that is extensively processed in the nucleus before being exported to the cytoplasm. Processing includes addition of a 5' cap (a methylated guanosine added to the 5' end, which protects the mRNA from degradation and aids in ribosome binding), polyadenylation (addition of a poly-A tail of 100–250 adenosine residues to the 3' end), and splicing (removal of non-coding intervening sequences called introns and joining of the coding exons).

Transfer RNA (tRNA) is the adapter molecule that translates the genetic code. Each tRNA molecule recognizes a specific three-nucleotide codon in mRNA through a complementary three-nucleotide anticodon sequence, and it carries the amino acid specified by that codon. The tRNA molecule is approximately 80 nucleotides long and folds into a characteristic cloverleaf secondary structure (four base-paired stems and three loops), which in three dimensions adopts an L-shaped tertiary structure. The anticodon loop is at one end of the L, and the 3' end where the amino acid is attached is at the other end.

Ribosomal RNA (rRNA) is the RNA component of ribosomes the molecular machines that synthesize all proteins. Ribosomes are enormous ribonucleoprotein complexes: the bacterial ribosome (70S) consists of a large subunit (50S) and a small subunit (30S), each containing rRNA molecules and dozens of proteins. Remarkably, it is the rRNA, not the protein component, that catalyzes the peptidyl transferase reaction the formation of peptide bonds during translation. This makes the ribosome a ribozyme an RNA catalyst a discovery that earned Thomas Cech and Sidney Altman the Nobel Prize in Chemistry in 1989.

Small nuclear RNAs (snRNAs) are a class of RNA found in the nucleus of eukaryotic cells. They associate with proteins to form snRNPs (small nuclear ribonucleoproteins, sometimes called snurps), which are the components of the spliceosome the giant molecular machine responsible for removing introns from pre-mRNA. The spliceosome is a ribozyme: the chemical steps of splicing are catalyzed by the snRNA components.

MicroRNAs (miRNAs) are small (approximately 22-nucleotide) RNA molecules that regulate gene expression by binding to complementary sequences in the 3' untranslated regions of mRNAs, causing their degradation or translational silencing. Humans encode over 2,000 miRNAs, and each miRNA can regulate hundreds of different mRNAs. miRNAs are involved in virtually every cellular process, from development and differentiation to immune responses and cancer. Aberrant miRNA expression is a hallmark of many cancers.

6.4 DNA Packaging: From Double Helix to Chromosome

The human genome contains approximately 3.2 billion base pairs of DNA a total length, if fully extended, of about 2 meters. Yet this DNA must be packaged into a nucleus that is typically only 5–10 micrometers in diameter. The compaction ratio is astonishing approximately 400,000-fold. And this packaging must be accomplished in a way that still allows the DNA to be read, copied, repaired, and regulated. The solution is an elaborate hierarchy of DNA folding called chromatin organization.

The first level of compaction involves nucleosomes the fundamental packaging unit of eukaryotic chromosomes. A nucleosome consists of approximately 147 base pairs of DNA wound 1.65 turns around a core of eight histone proteins (two each of histones H2A, H2B, H3, and H4). Histones are small, positively charged proteins that interact with the negatively charged phosphate backbone of DNA through electrostatic interactions. The core histone octamer acts as a molecular spool around which the DNA wraps tightly.

Nucleosomes are connected by short stretches of linker DNA (typically 10–50 base pairs), giving chromatin the appearance under the electron microscope of "beads on a string" a 10-nm fiber. Histone H1, a linker histone, binds to both the core particle and the linker DNA, stabilizing the 10-nm fiber.

The 10-nm fiber is further compacted into a 30-nm fiber a more tightly packed structure. The exact organization of the 30-nm fiber is still debated, but it involves the folding of the nucleosome chain into a compact, regular array.

Beyond the 30-nm fiber, chromatin is organized into loops domains of 50–100 kilobases of DNA attached to a protein scaffold. These loops are further organized into higher-order structures that ultimately give rise to the compact chromosomes visible under the light microscope during cell division. At the highest level of compaction (achieved at the metaphase stage of cell division), each chromosome is a densely packed structure of DNA, histone, and non-histone protein.

Crucially, chromatin structure is not static it is dynamically regulated in response to the cell's needs. Regions of active gene expression are typically found in open, accessible chromatin (euchromatin), while silenced regions tend to be more compact (heterochromatin). These states are regulated by chemical modifications of histone proteins (acetylation, methylation, phosphorylation, and more) and by ATP-dependent chromatin remodeling complexes that can slide, eject, or restructure nucleosomes. These regulatory processes constitute the field of epigenetics heritable changes in gene expression that do not involve changes in DNA sequence.

Chapter Summary

Nucleic acids are the information molecules of life the molecular libraries in which the instructions for building every protein and regulating every biological process are encoded. Nucleotides composed of a nitrogenous base, a pentose sugar, and a phosphate group are the monomers of DNA and RNA, linked by phosphodiester bonds into polymers with a defined 5'-to-3' directionality.

DNA adopts the iconic B-form double helix two antiparallel strands held together by Watson-Crick base pairing (A–T and G–C) and base stacking. This structure simultaneously stores genetic information (in the base sequence) and provides a mechanism for faithful copying (through complementary template-directed synthesis).

RNA is structurally similar to DNA but functionally far more diverse. mRNA carries genetic information from nucleus to cytoplasm. tRNA translates the genetic code. rRNA catalyzes peptide bond formation. snRNA participates in splicing. miRNA regulates gene expression. The RNA universe is vast and still being explored.

Eukaryotic DNA is packaged into nucleosomes 147 bp of DNA wrapped around histone octamers and organized into progressively higher levels of compaction, culminating in the mitotic chromosome. Chromatin structure is dynamically regulated by histone modifications and chromatin remodeling, governing which genes are accessible for transcription.

The next chapter explores how this genomic archive is faithfully copied the process of DNA replication.

CHAPTER 7

DNA Replication and Repair: Copying the Code of Life

Precision Machinery of Genome Duplication

Every time a cell divides, it must faithfully duplicate its entire genome billions of base pairs and distribute one complete copy to each daughter cell. In the human body, this happens roughly 3.8 million times every second. The entire genome of a human cell is replicated in the S phase of the cell cycle in approximately 8–10 hours. The machinery responsible for this replication must be extraordinarily fast, extraordinarily accurate, and extraordinarily well-regulated.

The accuracy of DNA replication is staggering. The overall error rate after proofreading and repair is approximately one mistake per 10 billion base pairs copied. To put this in perspective: if you were copying the text of this book at the same error rate, you could copy it ten thousand times before making a single mistake. This accuracy is not accidental it is the product of multiple overlapping mechanisms of error detection and correction, each adding another layer of fidelity to the replication process.

The key insight that guided the discovery of the replication mechanism was contained in the last sentence of the Watson-Crick double helix paper: if each strand serves as a template for the synthesis of a new complementary strand, then the two daughter molecules will each contain one original strand and one newly synthesized strand a mechanism called semiconservative replication. This prediction was brilliantly confirmed by Matthew Meselson and Franklin Stahl in 1958, in an experiment that has been called "the most beautiful experiment in biology."

7.1 The Semiconservative Model: Meselson and Stahl's Elegant Proof

In 1958, Matthew Meselson and Franklin Stahl devised an experiment of such clarity and elegance that it has become a classic of experimental biology. They grew E. coli bacteria for many generations in a medium containing ^{15}N-labeled ammonium chloride, allowing the heavy isotope of nitrogen to be incorporated into all nitrogenous bases of the bacteria's DNA. The DNA of these cells was uniformly "heavy" it contained ^{15}N in all base pairs.

They then transferred the bacteria to a medium containing only normal ^{14}N (light nitrogen) and allowed the cells to divide once, twice, and then multiple times. After each generation, they extracted the DNA and determined its density by equilibrium centrifugation in a cesium chloride density gradient a technique in which DNA molecules settle at a position in the gradient corresponding to their buoyant density.

The result was definitive. After one generation of growth in ^{14}N medium, all the DNA had an intermediate density exactly halfway between the pure ^{15}N density and the pure ^{14}N density. This could only be explained by semiconservative replication: each daughter molecule contained one ^{15}N strand (from the parent) and one new ^{14}N strand. After a second generation, half the DNA had intermediate density and half had light density — exactly as predicted if the two intermediate molecules each served as templates, with new ^{14}N strands synthesized on both strands.

This experiment ruled out two alternative models: conservative replication (in which both parental strands would remain together, generating one all-heavy and one all-light molecule after one generation) and dispersive replication (in which parental DNA would be fragmented and scattered randomly in both daughter molecules, generating a single intermediate-density band that would gradually lighten with successive generations). The semiconservative result was unambiguous.

7.2 The Replication Fork: An Assembly Line at the Molecular Scale

DNA replication begins at specific sequences in the genome called origins of replication sites where the double helix is first unwound and the replication machinery assembles. Bacteria typically have a single origin (oriC in E. coli), from which replication proceeds bidirectionally. Eukaryotic chromosomes, being far longer, have thousands of origins distributed along their length allowing simultaneous replication from many sites and completing the genome in hours rather than years.

At each origin, replication begins with the binding of initiator proteins that recognize and bind to the origin sequence. These proteins recruit additional factors that melt the DNA double helix (separate the two strands) at the origin, creating a replication bubble. From each end of the bubble, a replication fork moves outward as replication proceeds.

The replication fork is a site of remarkable complexity a molecular assembly line in which dozens of different proteins work in a precisely coordinated fashion. At the leading edge of the fork, a helicase enzyme (DnaB in bacteria; the MCM2–7 complex in eukaryotes) unwinds the DNA double helix by breaking the hydrogen bonds between base pairs and rotating the two strands apart. This unwinding is powered by ATP hydrolysis and proceeds at approximately 1,000 base pairs per second in bacteria.

Unwinding the helix ahead of the replication fork creates topological stress the DNA ahead becomes positively supercoiled as the two strands are forced apart. This stress is relieved by topoisomerases enzymes that transiently cut the DNA (one strand for type I topoisomerases, both strands for type II), allow rotation to relieve the stress, and then reseal the cut. Type II topoisomerases are the targets of important antibiotics (quinolones and fluoroquinolones, which trap the enzyme in a cut-DNA complex) and anti-cancer drugs (like the calprotectin's, which target eukaryotic topoisomerase I).

Single-strand DNA-binding proteins (SSBPs) bind to the separated strands at the fork, stabilizing them in the single-stranded state and preventing re-annealing (re-formation of the double helix) before they can be copied.

DNA synthesis is performed by DNA polymerase but this enzyme has two important limitations. First, it can only synthesize

DNA in the 5'-to-3' direction (it adds nucleotides to the 3'-OH end of the growing chain). Second, it cannot initiate a new chain from scratch it can only extend a pre-existing strand.

The first limitation creates the leading strand/lagging strand asymmetry that is one of the characteristic features of DNA replication. The leading strand is synthesized continuously in the direction of fork movement once initiated, the polymerase can synthesize continuously as the helicase unwinds the template ahead of it. The lagging strand is synthesized in the direction opposite to fork movement, requiring discontinuous synthesis: as the fork moves forward, the lagging strand template is periodically copied in short segments called Okazaki fragments (named after their discoverer, Reiji Okazaki), each of which is synthesized in the 5'-to-3' direction on a looped-back template.

7.3 DNA Polymerase: The Master Copier

DNA polymerase is the central enzyme of DNA replication the molecular machine that reads the template strand and synthesizes the complementary new strand. Understanding its mechanism reveals both the remarkable precision of DNA replication and the reasons for that precision.

DNA polymerase catalyzes a nucleophilic substitution reaction: the 3'-OH of the growing chain attacks the alpha-phosphate of the incoming deoxyribonucleoside triphosphate (dNTP), forming a new phosphodiester bond and releasing pyrophosphate (PPi). The subsequent hydrolysis of PPi to two phosphate ions by pyrophosphatase drives the reaction forward thermodynamically.

Before forming the bond, the polymerase checks whether the incoming dNTP is the correct complement of the template base. Incorrect nucleotides do not fit properly in the active site (which is shaped to accommodate only the correct Watson-Crick base pair) and are therefore incorporated at a far lower rate than correct ones. This initial selectivity gives a raw error rate of approximately 10^{-5} (one error per 100,000 nucleotides incorporated).

But DNA polymerase further reduces this error rate through a proofreading activity. Most DNA polymerases have a 3'-to-5' exonuclease activity the ability to remove nucleotides from the 3' end of the growing chain in addition to their 5'-to-3' polymerase activity. After each nucleotide incorporation, the polymerase pauses briefly to check whether the newly added nucleotide is correctly base-paired. If it is not, the mismatched nucleotide is removed by the exonuclease activity, and the correct nucleotide is incorporated. Proofreading reduces the error rate by another 100-fold, to approximately 10^{-7}.

After replication is complete, a final layer of error correction mismatch repair (MMR) scans the newly synthesized DNA for remaining base mismatches and corrects them. MMR reduces the final error rate to the extraordinary precision of approximately 10^{-10} per base pair one error per 10 billion nucleotides synthesized.

7.4 DNA Repair: Defending the Genome Against Damage

DNA replication errors are not the only threat to genomic integrity. The DNA of every cell is under constant assault from both endogenous and exogenous sources of damage. Reactive oxygen species (ROS) generated by cellular metabolism can oxidize bases and break the sugar-phosphate backbone. Spontaneous hydrolysis can remove bases (depurination) or deaminate cytosine to uracil. Environmental mutagens ultraviolet radiation, ionizing radiation, chemical carcinogens in tobacco smoke and industrial pollutants all damage DNA by creating a variety of base lesions and strand breaks. Estimates suggest that each human cell suffers between 10,000 and 1,000,000 DNA lesions per day.

Without repair, this damage would quickly accumulate to levels incompatible with normal cell function. To counter this threat, cells have evolved a sophisticated array of DNA repair pathways, each suited to repairing particular types of damage.

Base excision repair (BER) handles small, non-helix-distorting lesions damaged or inappropriate bases. It begins with a DNA glycosylase enzyme that recognizes and removes the damaged base, leaving an abasic site (AP site). An AP endonuclease then cuts the backbone at the AP site. DNA polymerase fills in the gap, and DNA ligase seals the nick. BER is responsible for correcting the thousands of oxidized and deaminated bases that arise in every cell every day.

Nucleotide excision repair (NER) handles bulky, helix-distorting lesions, particularly the pyrimidine dimers formed when UV light covalently links adjacent thymine (or cytosine) residues on the same DNA strand. NER works by cutting the damaged strand at two sites flanking the lesion, removing a short oligonucleotide of 25–30 bases, and filling in the gap using the undamaged complementary strand as template. The critical importance of NER is illustrated by xeroderma pigmentosum a rare inherited disease caused by mutations in NER genes. Patients with this condition are unable to repair UV-induced DNA damage and develop sunlight-induced skin cancers at extremely high rates.

Double-strand breaks (DSBs) in which both strands of the double helix are cut are the most dangerous type of DNA damage, as they can lead to chromosome fragmentation and translocation if not repaired. Two major pathways repair DSBs: non-homologous end joining (NHEJ), which directly ligates the broken ends (sometimes with small insertions or deletions at the junction), and homologous recombination (HR), which uses the sister chromatid or homologous chromosome as a template for precise repair. HR is error-free but requires a homologous template; NHEJ is faster but error-prone.

Chapter Summary

DNA replication is a semiconservative process each daughter molecule retains one parental strand and receives one newly synthesized complementary strand. Meselson and Stahl's experiment elegantly confirmed this model. Replication begins at origins of replication, where helicases unwind the double helix and the replication fork assembles.

DNA polymerase synthesizes new strands in the 5'-to-3' direction by extending pre-existing primers. The leading strand is synthesized continuously; the lagging strand is synthesized as discontinuous Okazaki fragments. Proofreading by the polymerase's 3'-to-5' exonuclease and post-replicative mismatch repair together achieve an error rate of approximately 10^{-10}.

DNA repair pathways base excision repair, nucleotide excision repair, and double-strand break repair defend the genome against the constant assault of endogenous and exogenous DNA-damaging agents. Failures of repair lead to mutation accumulation, which can cause cancer and premature aging.

In Chapter 8, we explore how the information stored in DNA is read and translated into the proteins that carry out all biological functions.

CHAPTER 8

Transcription and Translation: From Gene to Protein

Decoding the Central Dogma of Molecular Biology

Francis Crick articulated what he called the Central Dogma of molecular biology in 1958 a conceptual framework for understanding how genetic information flows in living systems. In its simplest form, the Central Dogma states: DNA makes RNA makes protein. Genetic information is stored in DNA, copied into RNA through a process called transcription, and then used to direct the synthesis of proteins through a process called translation.

This two-step process transcription followed by translation is universal to all cellular life. With the exception of RNA viruses (which store their genetic information in RNA and must first copy it to DNA before the cell can read it, using an enzyme called reverse transcriptase), all organisms use this same general strategy for gene expression.

The beauty of the central dogma is not merely that it describes information flow it is that it explains the logic of biological organization. DNA is the archive: stable, double-stranded, carefully protected, read-only. RNA is the working copy: transient, single-stranded, directly translated into protein. This division of labor makes evolutionary sense by keeping the archive separate from the working copies, cells can regulate which parts of the archive are read, and when, and how often, with great precision.

This chapter explores the molecular machinery and regulation of transcription and translation from the binding of RNA polymerase to promoter sequences, through the extraordinary choreography of the ribosome, to the diverse post-translational modifications that give proteins their final functional forms.

8.1 Transcription: Reading DNA Into RNA

Transcription is the process by which the information in a DNA sequence is copied into an RNA sequence. The enzyme responsible is RNA polymerase a large, multisubunit enzyme that reads the template (antisense) strand of DNA in the 3'-to-5' direction and synthesizes a complementary RNA strand in the 5'-to-3' direction. Unlike DNA polymerase, RNA polymerase does not require a primer it can initiate new RNA chains from scratch.

Transcription proceeds in three stages: initiation, elongation, and termination.

Initiation begins when RNA polymerase (or its eukaryotic equivalent, loaded via a complex of general transcription factors) binds to a specific DNA sequence called the promoter, located just upstream of the transcription start site. In bacteria, promoter recognition is mediated by the sigma factor a dissociable subunit of bacterial RNA polymerase that confers DNA-binding specificity. Different sigma factors recognize different promoter sequences, allowing bacteria to simultaneously regulate large sets of genes by changing which sigma factor is active.

Eukaryotic transcription is considerably more complex. Three distinct RNA polymerases handle different classes of RNA: RNA polymerase I synthesizes the large ribosomal RNAs, RNA polymerase II synthesizes mRNA and most non-coding RNAs (including snRNA and miRNA precursors), and RNA polymerase III synthesizes tRNA and the 5S ribosomal RNA. RNA polymerase II the most versatile and important requires a set of general transcription factors (TFIIA, TFIIB, TFIID, TFIIE, TFIIF, and TFIIH) to assemble at the promoter and position the polymerase correctly for initiation.

During elongation, RNA polymerase moves along the template strand, unwinding the DNA double helix ahead of it (creating a transcription bubble) and adding ribonucleotides to the growing RNA chain at a rate of approximately 20–50 nucleotides per second. Behind the polymerase, the DNA re-anneals (the two strands reform the double helix). The RNA chain peels off the template as it is synthesized, emerging as a single-stranded molecule.

Termination of transcription occurs at specific DNA sequences that signal the polymerase to stop. In bacteria, two main termination mechanisms operate: rho-independent termination, where the RNA transcript itself folds into a hairpin structure followed by a run of uridines that causes the polymerase to pause and dissociate, and rho-dependent termination, where the Rho protein (an ATP-dependent helicase) pursues the polymerase and dissociates it from the template when it catches up.

8.2 RNA Processing in Eukaryotes: From Pre-mRNA to Mature mRNA

In eukaryotes, the product of RNA polymerase II transcription is not directly usable as mRNA. The primary transcript called pre-mRNA or hnRNA (heterogeneous nuclear RNA) must undergo extensive processing in the nucleus before it can be exported to the cytoplasm and translated. This processing includes three major steps: 5' capping, 3' polyadenylation, and splicing.

5' capping occurs almost immediately after transcription begins. A 7-methylguanosine cap (m^7G cap) is added to the 5' end of the pre-mRNA through an unusual 5'-to-5' triphosphate linkage. The cap serves multiple functions: it protects the mRNA from degradation by 5' exonucleases, it signals that the RNA is a genuine mRNA (not an aberrant transcript), and it is recognized by translation initiation factors that recruit the ribosome to the mRNA.

3' polyadenylation occurs after the RNA polymerase transcribes past a polyadenylation signal (the hexanucleotide AAUAAA). This signal is recognized by a complex of proteins that cleave the nascent RNA approximately 15–30 nucleotides downstream and add a poly(A) tail of 200–250 adenosine residues. The poly(A) tail protects the 3' end of the mRNA from degradation, enhances translation efficiency, and plays a role in mRNA export from the nucleus.

Splicing is the most complex and remarkable of the three processing steps. Eukaryotic genes contain non-coding sequences called introns interspersed among the coding sequences (exons). These introns must be precisely removed from the pre-mRNA, and the flanking exons must be joined together, to produce a continuous coding sequence ready for translation. This is accomplished by the spliceosome — a giant molecular machine composed of five snRNPs (containing snRNA molecules U1, U2, U4, U5, and U6) and over 100 additional protein factors.

The spliceosome recognizes conserved sequences at the 5' and 3' splice sites flanking each intron and at a branch point within the intron. Through a series of two transesterification reactions, the intron is removed as a lariat structure (a loop) and the flanking exons are joined. The fidelity of splicing is extraordinary an error in a splice site can produce an aberrant protein or trigger nonsense-mediated decay (NMD), a cellular surveillance pathway that degrades mRNAs with premature stop codons.

Alternative splicing the inclusion or exclusion of different exons in different cell types, developmental stages, or physiological conditions dramatically expands the protein-coding capacity of the genome. The human genome contains approximately 20,000 protein-coding genes, yet the proteome (the full complement of proteins) contains an estimated 200,000–500,000 distinct protein forms. Most of this diversity is generated by alternative splicing.

8.3 The Genetic Code: Translation's Rosetta Stone

The genetic code is the set of rules by which the sequence of nucleotides in an mRNA is read by the ribosome and converted into a sequence of amino acids. The code was cracked between 1961 and 1966 through the combined efforts of several research groups an achievement often compared in difficulty and importance to the deciphering of the Egyptian hieroglyphics of the Rosetta Stone.

The genetic code is a triplet code: three consecutive nucleotides (a codon) specify one amino acid. With four possible nucleotides at each position, there are $4^3 = 64$ possible codons. Since there are only 20 amino acids to encode, plus signals for starting and stopping translation, the code is degenerate: most amino acids are encoded by more than one codon. Leucine, serine, and arginine each have six codons. Methionine and tryptophan each have only one. Three codons UAA, UAG, and UGA do not encode any amino acid but instead signal "stop" the end of the protein. One codon AUG (methionine) serves as the start codon for almost all proteins in all organisms.

The degeneracy of the genetic code is not random but structured: synonymous codons (codons that encode the same amino acid) typically differ only at the third position. This "wobble" at the third codon position first proposed by Francis Crick means that mutations at the third codon position often do not change the amino acid sequence (silent or synonymous mutations), and thus have no effect on the protein.

The genetic code is nearly universal with minor exceptions, the same codons specify the same amino acids in bacteria, archaea, plants, animals, and fungi. This universality is strong evidence that all life on Earth shares a common ancestor, and that the genetic code was established very early in the history of life. The few exceptions (mitochondria and certain ciliates use slightly different codes) represent rare evolutionary modifications from the universal code.

8.4 Translation: The Ribosome's Molecular Symphony

Translation is the process by which the ribosome reads the mRNA sequence (codon by codon) and builds a polypeptide chain (amino acid by amino acid). It is one of the most mechanically complex processes in biology, involving the coordinated action of the ribosome, dozens of translation factors, charged tRNA molecules, and the mRNA template.

Ribosomes are the factories of protein synthesis massive ribonucleoprotein assemblies (molecular weight approximately 2.5 MDa in bacteria) consisting of two subunits. The small subunit decodes the mRNA: it base-pairs codons in the mRNA with anticodons in tRNA molecules, checking that the correct tRNA is used. The large subunit catalyzes peptide bond formation and controls the movement of the ribosome along the mRNA. The interface between the two subunits contains three tRNA-binding sites: the A (aminoacyl) site, where the incoming charged tRNA binds; the P (peptidyl) site, where the growing polypeptide chain is held; and the E (exit) site, from which the deacylated tRNA leaves.

Translation begins with initiation, during which the ribosome assembles at the start codon (AUG) of the mRNA. The initiator tRNA (carrying methionine) binds to the P site of the ribosome positioned at the start codon. In bacteria, the ribosome is directed to the start codon by a ribosome-binding site (Shine-Dalgarno sequence) upstream of the AUG. In eukaryotes, the ribosome binds to the 5' cap and scans along the mRNA until it reaches the first AUG in a favorable context.

Elongation proceeds in a cyclic three-step mechanism: codon recognition (the correct aminoacyl-tRNA is delivered to the A site by elongation factor EF-Tu in bacteria, with GTP hydrolysis providing accuracy and energy), peptidyl transfer (the peptide chain in the P site is transferred to the amino group of the aminoacyl-tRNA in the A site, forming a new peptide bond catalyzed by the 23S rRNA of the large subunit), and translocation (the ribosome moves exactly three nucleotides along the mRNA, shifting the tRNAs from the A to P to E sites powered by GTP hydrolysis by elongation factor EF-G).

Elongation typically proceeds at a rate of 10–20 amino acids per second in bacteria and 3–5 per second in eukaryotes. A ribosome synthesizing a typical protein of 400 amino acids completes translation in under a minute. Multiple ribosomes often translate the same mRNA simultaneously, forming a polysome that maximizes the rate of protein production from a single mRNA molecule.

Chapter Summary

The Central Dogma DNA makes RNA makes protei describes the fundamental flow of genetic information in all cellular life. Transcription by RNA polymerase produces an RNA copy of each gene. In eukaryotes, the pre-mRNA is extensively processed: 5' capping, 3' polyadenylation, and splicing produce the mature mRNA that is exported to the cytoplasm.

The genetic code 64 triplet codons, 61 encoding amino acids plus 3 stop codons is degenerate and nearly universal. Translation by the ribosome converts the mRNA sequence into a polypeptide chain through three phases: initiation, elongation (codon recognition, peptidyl transfer, translocation), and termination. Post-translational modifications glycosylation, phosphorylation, ubiquitination, and many others give proteins their final functional states.

Having explored how genetic information is stored, copied, and expressed, we turn in Chapter 9 to how cells harvest and use energy the metabolic pathways that extract chemical energy from nutrients and use it to power all biological work.

CHAPTER 9

Metabolism: Energy Flow Through Biomolecules

Catabolism, Anabolism, and the Currency of Life

Life is fundamentally an energy-management operation. Every process that a living organism carries out moving, growing, responding, reproducing, even simply maintaining its molecular order against the constant tendency toward disorder requires a continuous input of energy. The ultimate source of nearly all this energy is sunlight, captured by photosynthetic organisms and stored in the chemical bonds of organic molecules. When animals eat plants (or eat animals that ate plants), they are recovering this stored solar energy through the controlled oxidation of biomolecules.

Metabolism is the totality of all chemical reactions in a cell the complete molecular operating system of life. It encompasses catabolism (the breaking down of molecules, with release of energy) and anabolism (the building up of molecules, with consumption of energy). These two processes are not independent the energy released by catabolism is captured and used to drive anabolism, creating an integrated, self-sustaining metabolic economy.

The central currency of this economy is ATP adenosine triphosphate. ATP is the molecule that captures the energy released by catabolic reactions (in the form of its high-energy phosphoanhydride bonds) and delivers that energy to anabolic reactions and other energy-requiring cellular processes. ATP is sometimes described as the "energy currency" of the cell, and this analogy is apt: just as money mediates exchanges between buyers and sellers without itself being the goods, ATP mediates energy exchanges between energy-releasing and energy-consuming reactions without itself being the ultimate energy source.

9.1 ATP: The Universal Energy Currency

Adenosine triphosphate (ATP) is a nucleotide the same class of molecule that makes up RNA and DNA consisting of adenosine (adenine base + ribose sugar) plus three phosphate groups linked in series. The three phosphate groups are called the alpha (α), beta (β), and gamma (γ) phosphates, from the one closest to the ribose outward. The bonds between the phosphate groups are phosphoanhydride bonds high-energy bonds whose hydrolysis releases significant amounts of free energy.

The hydrolysis of ATP to ADP (adenosine diphosphate) and inorganic phosphate (Pi) releases approximately -30.5 kJ/mol of free energy under standard conditions, and considerably more (approximately -50 kJ/mol) under physiological conditions (due to the low concentrations of ADP and Pi typically maintained in cells). This energy release is what makes ATP useful: it can be coupled to thermodynamically unfavorable (endergonic) reactions, making the combined reaction spontaneous.

But it would be a mistake to think of ATP simply as a "bag of energy" that is broken open when energy is needed. The mechanism by which ATP energy is coupled to biological work is specific and precise. In many cases, a phosphate group from ATP is transferred to another molecule (phosphorylation), activating it for a subsequent reaction. In other cases, the free energy of ATP hydrolysis drives a conformational change in a motor protein or ion pump, performing mechanical or osmotic work.

The cellular concentration of ATP is carefully regulated and maintained at approximately 1–5 mM. Because ATP is consumed continuously by the cell, it must be continuously regenerated. The adult human body turns over its own weight in ATP every day the amount of ATP in the body at any given moment is only about 40 grams, but this pool is recycled thousands of times per day through ADP rephosphorylation. The pathways that regenerate ATP glycolysis, the citric acid cycle, and oxidative phosphorylation are therefore among the most important and most carefully regulated pathways in all of biochemistry.

9.2 Glycolysis: Ten Steps to Energy

Glycolysis is the ancient, universal pathway by which glucose is partially oxidized to pyruvate. It occurs in the cytoplasm of all cells bacteria, archaea, fungi, plants, and animals and requires no oxygen. It is the foundation upon which all more elaborate energy metabolism is built.

The word "glycolysis" comes from the Greek words for "sweet" (glykys) and "loosening" (lysis), capturing the idea of breaking apart sugar. The pathway consists of ten sequential enzyme-catalyzed reactions that transform one molecule of glucose (6 carbons) into two molecules of pyruvate (3 carbons each), with a net production of 2 ATP and 2 NADH.

The pathway can be conceptually divided into two phases. The investment phase (first five reactions) uses 2 ATP molecules to phosphorylate glucose and split it into two three-carbon units. The payoff phase (last five reactions) oxidizes these three-carbon units and generates 4 ATP and 2 NADH for a net gain of 2 ATP.

The first step, catalyzed by hexokinase, phosphorylates glucose at carbon-6 using one ATP. This serves two purposes: it traps glucose inside the cell (phosphorylated glucose cannot cross the cell membrane) and begins the process of activating glucose for subsequent reactions. In the liver, the equivalent reaction is catalyzed by glucokinase (hexokinase IV), which has a much higher Km for glucose and is not inhibited by glucose-6-phosphateproperties that make it a sensor of blood glucose levels rather than a steady-state catalyst.

The rate-limiting step of glycolysis the point of greatest regulatory control is the reaction catalyzed by phosphofructokinase-1 (PFK-1), which adds a second phosphate group to fructose-6-phosphate to produce fructose-1,6-bisphosphate. PFK-1 is a classic allosteric enzyme, regulated by the energy status of the cell: it is inhibited by ATP (high energy status signals that less glycolysis is needed) and by citrate (an indicator that the citric acid cycle is well-supplied), and activated by AMP and ADP (low energy status signals) and fructose-2,6-bisphosphate (a potent activator controlled by hormonal signals).

The net yield of glycolysi 2 ATP and 2 NADH per glucose is modest. The pyruvate produced still contains most of the chemical energy of the original glucose molecule. Under aerobic conditions, pyruvate is transported into the mitochondrion and oxidized completely to CO_2 through the citric acid cycle and oxidative phosphorylation, generating an additional 30–32 ATP per glucose. Under anaerobic conditions (when oxygen is limited), pyruvate is instead reduced to lactate (in animals) or ethanol and CO_2 (in yeast) reactions that regenerate NAD+ from NADH, allowing glycolysis to continue.

9.3 The Citric Acid Cycle: The Central Hub of Metabolism

The citric acid cycle also called the Krebs cycle, after its discoverer Hans Krebs, or the tricarboxylic acid (TCA) cycle is the central metabolic hub of aerobic organisms. It is not merely a pathway for glucose oxidation: it is the common oxidative pathway for all major fuels carbohydrates, fatty acids, and amino acids all of which are ultimately converted to acetyl-CoA (or directly to cycle intermediates) before entering the cycle.

The cycle begins when acetyl-CoA (two-carbon unit) condenses with oxaloacetate (four-carbon compound) to form citrate (six-carbon). Over the course of eight reactions, citrate is progressively oxidized. Two carbon atoms are lost as CO_2 (balancing the two carbons that entered as acetyl-CoA), and the cycle regenerates oxaloacetate ready to accept another acetyl-CoA and begin again.

The energetic yield per turn of the cycle is substantial: 3 NADH, 1 $FADH_2$, 1 GTP (equivalent to 1 ATP), and 2 CO_2. These electron carriers NADH and $FADH_2$ carry the electrons stripped from the oxidized carbon compounds to the electron transport chain, where their oxidation drives the synthesis of the bulk of the cell's ATP.

But the citric acid cycle does far more than produce electron carriers for ATP synthesis. Its intermediates are the starting materials for numerous biosynthetic pathways. Oxaloacetate is the precursor of aspartate and asparagine. Alpha-ketoglutarate gives rise to glutamate and glutamine, the principal amino group donors for the synthesis of all other amino acids. Succinyl-CoA is the precursor of porphyrins the ring structures of heme and chlorophyll. Citrate provides acetyl-CoA for fatty acid synthesis in the cytoplasm. In this role as both a catabolic and biosynthetic hub, the citric acid cycle exemplifies the interconnectedness of metabolism the reason why disrupting one metabolic pathway often has cascading effects on many others.

9.4 Oxidative Phosphorylation: The Powerhouse Within the Powerhouse

The majority of ATP synthesis in aerobic organisms is accomplished not by glycolysis or the citric acid cycle directly, but by a process called oxidative phosphorylation the coupling of electron transport through the inner mitochondrial membrane to the phosphorylation of ADP to ATP.

The electron transport chain (ETC) consists of four large protein complexes (Complexes I, II, III, and IV) embedded in the inner mitochondrial membrane. Electrons from NADH and

$FADH_2$ the electron carriers produced by glycolysis and the citric acid cycle are passed sequentially through these complexes, ultimately being delivered to molecular oxygen (O_2) at Complex IV (cytochrome c oxidase), where they combine with protons to form water. This is why aerobic organisms require oxygen: it is the final electron acceptor of the ETC, without which the entire chain would stall.

As electrons move from Complex I to Complex IV, they flow spontaneously from compounds of higher electron potential to those of lower potential "downhill" in energy terms. The energy released by this electron flow is captured and used to pump protons (H^+) from the matrix of the mitochondrion across the inner membrane into the intermembrane space. This proton pumping creates an electrochemical gradient a combination of concentration gradient and electrical potential known as the proton-motive force (PMF).

The PMF is the immediate energy source for ATP synthase (Complex V) the remarkable molecular turbine that synthesizes ATP. Protons flow back into the mitochondrial matrix through the ATP synthase, moving "downhill" along their electrochemical gradient, and this flow drives the rotation of the rotor component of ATP synthase. This rotation drives conformational changes in the catalytic head of the enzyme that couple ADP + Pi binding with ATP synthesis and release. The chemiosmotic mechanism for ATP synthesis proposed by Peter Mitchell in 1961, for which he received the Nobel Prize is one of the most elegant and important concepts in all of biochemistry.

The overall yield of complete oxidation of one glucose molecule glycolysis + pyruvate dehydrogenase + citric acid cycle + oxidative phosphorylation is approximately 30–32 ATP. The efficiency of this conversion is remarkably high, approximately 40%, compared to the typical 25–35% efficiency of internal combustion engines.

Chapter Summary

Metabolism is the integrated network of chemical reactions that sustains life. ATP, synthesized by substrate-level phosphorylation and oxidative phosphorylation, is the universal energy currency. Glycolysis breaks glucose into pyruvate with a net yield of 2 ATP and 2 NADH. The citric acid cycle oxidizes acetyl-CoA completely to CO_2, generating NADH and $FADH_2$. Oxidative phosphorylation couple's electron transport through the ETC to proton pumping, and the resulting proton-motive force drives ATP synthase to produce the bulk of the cell's ATP.

Fatty acid beta-oxidation in the mitochondrion provides a second major fuel source, generating acetyl-CoA, NADH, and $FADH_2$ from fatty acid chains. Gluconeogenesis in the liver replenishes blood glucose during fasting. The integration of these pathways ensures that the cell's energy needs are met across varying nutritional states.

CHAPTER 10

Biomolecular Interactions: Communication and Signaling

How Molecules Talk to Each Other Inside the Cell

A living cell is not simply a bag of enzymes randomly catalyzing reactions. It is a highly organized, exquisitely responsive system that must continuously monitor its environment, coordinate the activities of thousands of molecular machines, adjust its behavior in response to changing conditions, and communicate with neighboring cells in a multicellular organism. All of this coordination depends on molecular communication the ability of one molecule to convey information to another.

Biomolecular communication operates at every scale, from the binding of a substrate in an enzyme's active site (communication within a single protein) to the binding of a hormone to a surface receptor (communication between organs across vast physiological distances). The principles that govern all these interactions are the same: molecules bind to each other through non-covalent forces with a specificity determined by their complementary shapes and charge distributions, and this binding alters the properties of one or both partners triggering a cascade of downstream events.

Understanding cell signaling the molecular language by which cells respond to their environment is not merely academic. The dysregulation of signaling pathways is a central feature of cancer, diabetes, autoimmune diseases, neurological disorders, and many other diseases. And the manipulation of signaling pathways by drugs that mimic or block specific molecular interactions is one of the most productive strategies of modern pharmacology.

10.1 Non-Covalent Forces: The Molecular Grammar of Signaling

All biological recognition event the binding of a hormone to its receptor, an enzyme to its substrate, an antibody to its antigen, a transcription factor to its DNA binding site are mediated by non-covalent forces. These forces are individually weak (each contributing only 1–10 kJ/mol of binding energy), but they act collectively, with many forces operating simultaneously between two complementary surfaces, to create tight and specific binding interactions.

Hydrogen bonds form when a hydrogen atom covalently bonded to an electronegative atom (O or N) is attracted to another electronegative atom on a neighboring molecule. In biological recognition, hydrogen bonds provide both energy and specificity: only molecules that can form complementary hydrogen bonding patterns will bind to each other with high affinity. The AT and GC base pairs of the DNA double helix are stabilized by 2 and 3 hydrogen bonds, respectively. Enzyme-substrate interactions, antibody-antigen recognition, and receptor-hormone binding all depend critically on networks of hydrogen bonds.

Electrostatic interactions (ionic bonds) occur between oppositely charged groups for example, between a positively charged lysine side chain and a negatively charged phosphate group. These interactions are strong at short range but diminish with distance. Salt bridges in the interior of proteins and at protein-protein interfaces are important contributors to binding specificity and stability.

The hydrophobic effect, as discussed in previous chapters, drives the burial of hydrophobic surfaces when molecules associate in aqueous solution. When a ligand binds to a protein, the hydrophobic portions of the binding interface are sequestered from water, providing a powerful thermodynamic driving force for association. Approximately half of the binding energy in protein-ligand interactions comes from the hydrophobic effect.

Van der Waals forces are extremely short-range (falling off as the sixth power of distance) attractive interactions between any two adjacent atoms due to transient fluctuations in electron distribution. They are individually tiny but collectively important when two large surfaces are in close contact. The precise fit of a substrate in an enzyme's active site the "snugness" of the fit is largely determined by van der Waals complementarity between the surfaces.

The dissociation constant (Kd) is the quantitative measure of binding affinity between two molecules. It is defined as the concentration of ligand at which half the binding sites are occupied. A low Kd indicates tight binding (high affinity); a high Kd indicates loose binding (low affinity). The Kd of a high-affinity hormone-receptor pair might be in the picomolar range (10^{-12} M), while a low-affinity interaction might have a Kd in the millimolar range (10^{-3} M). The extraordinary range of binding affinities available through non-covalent interactions spanning over nine orders of magnitude allows biological systems to fine-tune the threshold and duration of molecular recognition events with exquisite precision.

10.2 G Protein-Coupled Receptors: Masters of Signal Transduction

G protein-coupled receptors (GPCRs) are the largest family of cell surface receptors in the human genome, with approximately 800 members. They mediate the cellular responses to an extraordinary diversity of extracellular signals hormones, neurotransmitters, odorants, light (through the visual pigment rhodopsin), tastants, and many drugs. Over 30% of all currently approved drugs target GPCRs, making this family of proteins the most important class of drug targets in the pharmaceutical industry.

All GPCRs share a common structural feature: a single polypeptide chain that threads through the cell membrane seven times (hence they are also called seven-transmembrane receptors or serpentine receptors). The extracellular loops and the N-terminus form the ligand-binding domain. The intracellular loops and C-terminus interact with heterotrimeric G proteins (composed of Gα, Gβ, and Gγ subunits) on the cytoplasmic face of the membrane.

When a ligand binds to the extracellular face of a GPCR, it induces a conformational change that propagates through the transmembrane helices to the intracellular face, where it activates the associated G protein. Activation involves the exchange of GDP for GTP on the Gα subunit, causing Gα to dissociate from Gβγ. Both Gα-GTP and Gβγ can then activate or inhibit downstream effectors enzymes or ion channels.

The Gα subunit has intrinsic GTPase activity it hydrolyzes GTP to GDP + Pi on its own, turning itself off and allowing reassociation with Gβγ. The rate of this self-inactivation can be modulated by RGS proteins (regulators of G protein signaling), which accelerate GTP hydrolysis and are important regulatory elements of GPCR signaling.

Through these downstream effectors, GPCR activation generates second messengers small, diffusible intracellular signaling molecules that amplify and distribute the signal throughout the cell. The classic GPCR second messenger is cyclic AMP (cAMP), produced from ATP by the enzyme adenylyl cyclase when activated by Gαs. cAMP binds to and activates protein kinase A (PKA), which then phosphorylates numerous target proteins, altering their activity. This amplification cascade means that the binding of a single hormone molecule to a single receptor can activate thousands of PKA molecules, which in turn can phosphorylate hundreds of thousands of target proteins a remarkable amplification of the original signal.

10.3 Receptor Tyrosine Kinases: Growth Factor Signaling

While GPCRs are the most numerous classes of cell surface receptors, receptor tyrosine kinases (RTKs) are arguably the most important regulators of cell growth, proliferation, differentiation, and survival. Their dysregulation is a central feature of virtually every human cancer.

RTKs are transmembrane proteins with an extracellular ligand-binding domain, a single transmembrane helix, and an intracellular kinase domain. Ligands for RTKs are typically growth factors small proteins that promote cell growth and division. Upon ligand binding, RTKs undergo dimerization (two receptor molecules come together), which activates their intracellular kinase domains. The activated kinase domains cross-phosphorylate each other on multiple tyrosine residues (autophosphorylation), creating docking sites for intracellular signaling proteins.

These phosphotyrosine docking sites recruit adaptor proteins and signaling enzymes that recognize them through specialized phosphotyrosine-binding domains (SH2 domains, PTB domains). The recruited proteins in turn activate downstream signaling pathways including the RAS/MAP kinase pathway (promoting cell proliferation), the PI3K/AKT pathway (promoting cell survival and growth), and the STAT pathway (regulating gene expression).

The EGF receptor (EGFR, epidermal growth factor receptor) is a prototypical RTK and one of the most important cancer drug targets. Mutations that constitutively activate EGFR keeping it active even without EGF binding are found in many lung cancers. Drugs like gefitinib and erlotinib, which inhibit EGFR's kinase activity, have transformed the treatment of EGFR-mutant lung cancers.

10.4 Second Messengers: Amplifying the Signal

Second messengers are small, rapidly diffusible intracellular molecules that are generated in response to extracellular signals and serve to amplify and distribute those signals throughout the cell. The concept of second messengers introduced by Earl Sutherland, who won the Nobel Prize for his work on cAMP revolutionized our understanding of cellular signaling.

Cyclic AMP (cAMP) was the first second messenger to be identified. Produced from ATP by adenylyl cyclase (activated by Gαs-coupled receptors), cAMP diffuses rapidly through the cytoplasm and activates protein kinase A (PKA) by binding to its regulatory subunits and releasing its catalytic subunits. PKA phosphorylates enzymes, transcription factors, and structural proteins on serine and threonine residues, altering their activities. cAMP is broken down by phosphodiesterase enzymes (PDEs), which are important drug targets: Viagra (sildenafil) works by inhibiting a PDE specific for cyclic GMP (cGMP), prolonging the signaling of nitric oxide in vascular smooth muscle.

Calcium (Ca^{2+}) is arguably the most versatile and important second messenger in biology. Cytoplasmic calcium concentration is kept extremely low at rest (approximately 100 nM) by active transport of Ca^{2+} out of the cytoplasm (into the extracellular space or the ER lumen). When signaling pathways generate IP3 (inositol trisphosphate), it binds to IP3 receptors in the ER membrane and triggers Ca^{2+} release into the cytoplasm. Cytoplasmic Ca^{2+} can rise 10–100-fold in a matter of milliseconds, providing a rapid and dramatic signal.

Calcium signals are decoded by calcium-binding proteins, most prominently calmodulin a small, dumbbell-shaped protein with four Ca^{2+}-binding sites. When saturated with Ca^{2+}, calmodulin undergoes a conformational change that allows it to bind and activate a wide variety of target enzymes and proteins, including calmodulin-dependent kinases (CaMKs), which in turn phosphorylate numerous downstream targets. This calcium-calmodulin signaling axis controls muscle contraction, neurotransmitter release, gene expression, and many other biological processes.

Chapter Summary

Cell signaling depends on molecular recognition the binding of signaling molecules (ligands) to their receptors through non-covalent forces. G protein-coupled receptors, the largest family of drug targets, activate heterotrimeric G proteins that generate second messengers (cAMP, Ca^{2+}, DAG) and propagate signals through kinase cascades. Receptor tyrosine kinases mediate growth factor signaling and regulate cell proliferation, survival, and differentiation their dysregulation drives cancer.

Second messengers amplify and distribute signals, allowing single ligand-receptor binding events to alter the activities of thousands of target proteins. The reversibility of these signaling events through GTPases, phosphatases, and second-messenger-degrading enzymes ensures that signals are transient and precisely controlled.

Chapter 11 explores how disruptions of biomolecular function lead to disease, and how understanding biomolecules at the molecular level has opened revolutionary new avenues for therapy.

CHAPTER 11

Biomolecules in Disease and Medicine

From Molecular Pathology to Therapeutic Targets

Modern medicine has been transformed by a simple but profound insight: diseases are, at their most fundamental level, disorders of molecules. Cancer is not merely uncontrolled cell growth — it is the consequence of specific mutations in specific genes that encode specific proteins, altering their activity in specific ways. Diabetes is not merely high blood sugar — it is the failure of specific molecular signaling pathways involving insulin, its receptor, and the downstream kinases and glucose transporters that mediate the cellular response to insulin. Alzheimer's disease is not merely memory loss — it is the aggregation of specific proteins into specific fibrillar structures that disrupt neuronal function in specific brain regions.

This molecular understanding of disease has two immediate practical implications. First, it allows us to diagnose disease with unprecedented precision to identify the specific molecular lesion responsible for a patient's condition and predict its likely course. Second, it opens the door to targeted therapy the design of drugs that interact with the specific molecular abnormality responsible for a disease, rather than the broader, less specific interventions of earlier medicine.

The story of molecular medicine is one of the most exciting narratives in modern science a story of conceptual revolutions, technological breakthroughs, and life-saving applications. This chapter explores several of the most important intersections between biomolecular science and human disease.

11.1 Protein Misfolding Diseases: When Proteins Go Astray

The correct three-dimensional structure of a protein is not merely desirable it is essential for function. When proteins misfold adopting incorrect, non-native conformations the consequences can range from simple loss of function to the formation of toxic protein aggregates that damage and kill cells.

Alzheimer's disease is the most common neurodegenerative disorder, affecting approximately 50 million people worldwide. At its molecular core lie two types of abnormal protein deposits: amyloid plaques (extracellular aggregates of amyloid-beta peptide) and neurofibrillary tangles (intracellular aggregates of hyperphosphorylated tau protein). Amyloid-beta is a 40–42 amino acid peptide generated by proteolytic cleavage of the amyloid precursor protein (APP). In Alzheimer's disease, this peptide misfolds and aggregates into oligomers and fibrils characterized by a cross-beta sheet structure in which beta strands run perpendicular to the fibril axis, creating a ladder-like arrangement of hydrogen bonds along the fibril length. Current therapeutic strategies targeting amyloid-beta include antibodies that clear amyloid deposits, inhibitors of the secretases that generate amyloid-beta, and inhibitors of amyloid fibril formation.

Parkinson's disease is characterized by the death of dopaminergic neurons in the substantia nigra, leading to the motor symptoms of tremor, rigidity, and slowness of movement. The molecular signature of Parkinson's is the Lewy body an intracellular inclusion body consisting primarily of aggregated alpha-synuclein protein. Alpha-synuclein is normally a small, soluble protein associated with synaptic vesicles. In Parkinson's disease, it misfolds and aggregates into oligomers and fibrils. Mutations in alpha-synuclein cause rare familial forms of Parkinson's, and even normal alpha-synuclein can aggregate in response to certain environmental conditions and genetic risk factors.

Prion diseases represent perhaps the most philosophically challenging protein misfolding disorders: they are transmissible they can spread from organism to organism but the infectious agent is not a virus, bacterium, or nucleic acid. It is a protein. Prion diseases (including scrapie in sheep, bovine spongiform encephalopathy "mad cow disease" in cattle, Creutzfeldt-Jakob disease in humans, and chronic wasting disease in deer) are caused by the prion protein (PrP) adopting an abnormal conformation. The misfolded form (PrPSc) is resistant to proteolysis and can induce the normal form (PrPC) to misfold acting as a template for its own propagation.

11.2 Cancer at the Molecular Level: Oncogenes and Tumor Suppressors

Cancer is ultimately a disease of DNA specifically, of the accumulation of mutations in genes that regulate cell growth, division, death, and differentiation. Normal cells replicate in a carefully controlled manner; cancer cells escape this control and divide indefinitely, invading surrounding tissues and spreading to distant sites (metastasis). Understanding cancer requires understanding the molecular machinery of cell cycle control and the specific ways in which mutations subvert that machinery.

Proto-oncogenes are normal cellular genes that encode proteins promoting cell growth and division growth factors, growth factor receptors, signal transduction proteins, and transcription factors. When mutated (or amplified, or abnormally activated) to create oncogenes, these genes drive excessive cell proliferation. The RAS family of GTPases are among the most commonly mutated oncogenes in human cancers: mutations in KRAS, NRAS, or HRAS are found in approximately 25% of all human tumors. Oncogenic RAS mutations lock RAS in the GTP-bound (active) state by impairing its GTPase activity, resulting in constitutive activation of growth-promoting downstream pathways regardless of whether growth factor receptors are occupied.

Tumor suppressor genes, by contrast, encode proteins that restrain cell division or promote cell death. Loss of function of tumor suppressors through mutation, deletion, or epigenetic silencing removes these brakes on cell proliferation. TP53, encoding the p53 protein, is the most frequently mutated gene in human cancers: mutations in TP53 are found in approximately

50% of all tumors. The p53 protein acts as a "guardian of the genome" it is activated by DNA damage and other cellular stresses, and it can arrest the cell cycle (allowing time for repair), activate DNA repair, or trigger apoptosis (programmed cell death) if the damage is irreparable. Loss of p53 allows cells to divide despite genomic damage, dramatically accelerating the accumulation of additional cancer-promoting mutations.

The era of targeted cancer therapy began with imatinib (Gleevec), a drug designed to inhibit the BCR-ABL fusion kinase that drives chronic myelogenous leukemia (CML). BCR-ABL arises from a chromosomal translocation that fuses the BCR gene to the ABL tyrosine kinase gene, creating a constitutively active kinase. Imatinib fits into the ATP-binding pocket of BCR-ABL and blocks its activity, converting a previously fatal diagnosis into a manageable chronic condition for most patients. The success of imatinib demonstrated the power of targeted molecular therapy and launched the modern era of cancer pharmacogenomics.

11.3 Drug Design: The Art of Molecular Targeting

The ultimate application of understanding biomolecules at the structural level is rational drug design the creation of molecules that interact with specific biological targets in specific ways to achieve a desired therapeutic effect. Modern drug design has been transformed by advances in structural biology (X-ray crystallography, NMR, cryo-electron microscopy), computational chemistry, and high-throughput screening.

The starting point for drug design is the target a specific biomolecule (usually a protein, but increasingly nucleic acids and even protein-protein interactions) whose activity is abnormal in a disease state and whose modulation would provide therapeutic benefit. Once a target is identified and validated, the drug designer seeks molecules called lead compounds that bind to the target with sufficient affinity and selectivity.

Structure-based drug design uses the three-dimensional structure of the target (typically determined by X-ray crystallography or cryo-EM) to guide the design or modification of lead compounds. By visualizing the exact geometry of the binding site and the interactions between a lead compound and the target, medicinal chemists can rationally modify the compound's structure to improve its potency, selectivity, pharmacokinetics, and drug-like properties.

Monoclonal antibodies represent a different class of targeted therapy. These are large protein molecules (immunoglobulins) produced by a single clone of B cells that recognize a specific antigen with high affinity and selectivity. Since the development of hybridoma technology by Köhler and Milstein in 1975 (for which they received the Nobel Prize), monoclonal antibodies have become major therapeutic agents particularly in oncology, autoimmune disease, and inflammatory conditions. Trastuzumab (Herceptin), which targets the HER2 receptor overexpressed in certain breast cancers; rituximab, which targets the CD20 protein on B cells for treatment of B cell lymphoma; and adalimumab (Humira), which neutralizes TNF-alpha in rheumatoid arthritis and Crohn's disease are among the most successful therapeutic molecules ever developed.

11.4 CRISPR-Cas9: Rewriting the Biomolecular Blueprint

In 2012, Jennifer Doudna, Emmanuelle Charpentier, and their collaborators published a paper that would transform biology: they showed that a bacterial immune system component the Cas9 protein guided by a small RNA molecule could be programmed to cut DNA at any desired sequence with extraordinary precision. CRISPR-Cas9 gene editing was born, and in 2020, Doudna and Charpentier were awarded the Nobel Prize in Chemistry.

CRISPR (Clustered Regularly Interspaced Short Palindromic Repeats) is a component of the adaptive immune system of bacteria. When bacteria survive a viral infection, they incorporate short sequences of the viral DNA into their own genome, in a region of the bacterial chromosome flanked by repetitive sequences the CRISPR array. If the same virus attacks again, these stored sequences are transcribed into small RNA molecules (crRNAs) that guide the Cas9 protein to the matching viral DNA, which Cas9 then cleaves destroying the virus.

The genius of the CRISPR-Cas9 system is its programmability. By changing the sequence of the guide RNA (gRNA), the complex can be directed to cut any target DNA sequence of the form 5'-N_{20}-NGG-3' (where N is any nucleotide and NGG is the PAM protospacer adjacent motif — required for Cas9 binding). This sequence requirement is met roughly every 8–10 base pairs in the human genome, giving extraordinary flexibility in target choice.

CRISPR-Cas9 has been used to correct disease-causing mutations in cultured cells and animal models of numerous genetic diseases, including sickle cell disease, Duchenne muscular dystrophy, and cystic fibrosis. In December 2023, the FDA approved the first two CRISPR-based therapies: Casgevy and Lyfgenia, for the treatment of sickle cell disease marking a historic milestone in the translation of gene editing from concept to clinical reality.

Beyond simple gene disruption, CRISPR tools have been extended in numerous ways: base editors can change single DNA bases without cutting both strands of the DNA; prime editors can make small insertions, deletions, and all twelve types of point mutations; CRISPRi and CRISPRa can repress or activate gene expression without altering the DNA sequence. The pace of CRISPR innovation shows no sign of slowing.

Chapter Summary

Diseases are molecular disorders the consequence of specific disruptions in the structure, function, or regulation of biomolecules. Protein misfolding diseases (Alzheimer's, Parkinson's, prion diseases) arise from the aggregation of misfolded proteins into toxic amyloid-like structures. Cancer results from the accumulation of mutations in proto-oncogenes and tumor suppressor genes that regulate cell cycle progression and apoptosis. Molecular targeting by small-molecule drugs and monoclonal antibodies has transformed the treatment of many cancers and inflammatory diseases.

CRISPR-Cas9 gene editing has opened the era of precise genomic medicine, with the first FDA-approved CRISPR-based therapies now in clinical use. The pace of translation from biomolecular discovery to therapeutic application has never been faster.

The final chapter looks to the future to the emerging frontiers of biomolecular science where today's basic research is laying the foundation for tomorrow's transformative technologies.

CHAPTER 12

Frontiers in Biomolecular Science

Emerging Technologies and the Future of Life Sciences

The history of biomolecular science is a history of revolutions. The discovery of the double helix was a revolution. The cracking of the genetic code was a revolution. The development of recombinant DNA technology was a revolution. The polymerase chain reaction was a revolution. Each of these transformative discoveries built on the preceding ones, and each opened new questions, new technologies, and new possibilities that its discoverers could barely have imagined.

We are living through another such revolutionary period arguably the most fertile and rapidly advancing era in the history of the life sciences. Technologies that were theoretical just a decade ago are now routine. Diseases that were death sentences a generation ago are now manageable, or even curable. And on the horizon are capabilities the ability to read and write the entire genomes of organisms, to design proteins from scratch, to cure genetic diseases in living patients, to construct entirely new forms of life that raise not only scientific questions but profound ethical ones.

This final chapter surveys the most exciting frontiers of biomolecular science as of the mid-2020s: the omics revolution, synthetic biology, nanobiotechnology, artificial intelligence in drug discovery, and the ethical dimensions of these technologies. It is, of necessity, a snapshot of a rapidly moving field by the time you read this, some of what is described as cutting-edge may already be standard practice.

12.1 The Omics Revolution: Biology at the Systems Level

For most of its history, biochemistry and molecular biology were inherently reductionist sciences they studied one molecule, one pathway, one gene at a time. This approach produced extraordinary knowledge, but it also had an inherent limitation: cells do not operate one molecule at a time. They operate as integrated systems in which thousands of molecules interact simultaneously, and the behavior of the system cannot always be predicted from the properties of the individual components.

The omics revolution the development of technologies capable of measuring entire classes of biomolecules simultaneously and comprehensively has given biologists a systems-level view of cellular function for the first time.

Genomics is the large-scale analysis of genomes entire DNA sequences of organisms. The Human Genome Project, completed in 2003, sequenced the complete human genome at a cost of approximately 3 billion dollars over 13 years. Today, a human genome can be sequenced in a few hours at a cost of under $500.

This 10-million-fold reduction in cost and time has been driven by next-generation sequencing (NGS) technologies, which sequence millions of DNA fragments simultaneously in massively parallel reactions. Clinical genomics the routine sequencing of patients' genomes to guide diagnosis and treatment is rapidly becoming standard medical practice.

Transcriptomics measures the complete set of RNA molecules (the transcriptome) in a cell or tissue at a given time, providing a snapshot of gene expression. RNA-seq (RNA sequencing) has replaced the earlier microarray technology as the standard method for transcriptome analysis. Single-cell RNA sequencing (scRNA-seq) allows the transcriptome of each individual cell in a heterogeneous tissue to be measured separately revealing cellular diversity and dynamics that are invisible in bulk measurements.

Proteomics measures the complete complement of proteins (the proteome) in a cell or tissue. Mass spectrometry is the primary technology of proteomics: proteins are digested into peptides, which are separated by their mass-to-charge ratio and identified by comparison to protein databases. Modern proteomic approaches can detect and quantify thousands of proteins simultaneously, including their post-translational modifications.

Metabolomics measures the small-molecule metabolites in a biological sample the end products and intermediates of metabolism. Metabolomics provides the most direct readout of the cell's current functional state, reflecting not just which genes are expressed (genomics, transcriptomics) or which proteins are present (proteomics) but what those proteins are actually doing.

The integration of data from multiple omics levels multi-omics is the frontier of systems biology. By combining genomic, transcriptomic, proteomic, and metabolomic data from the same biological system, researchers can build comprehensive molecular models of cellular function, identify disease biomarkers, and discover new therapeutic targets.

12.2 Synthetic Biology: Engineering Life

Synthetic biology applies the principles of engineering to biological systems designing and constructing new biological parts, devices, and systems that do not exist in nature, or redesigning existing biological systems for new purposes. It is the logical extension of our ability to read and write genetic information: if we can sequence genomes and edit them, why not design entirely new ones?

The field began with the construction of simple genetic "parts" standardized, modular genetic elements (promoters, ribosome binding sites, coding sequences, terminators) that could be combined like electronic components to build genetic circuits. The Registry of Standard Biological Parts, begun at MIT, catalogued thousands of such parts and made them available to researchers worldwide. Teams of undergraduate students compete annually in the IGEM (International Genetically Engineered Machine) competition to design novel biological systems from these parts.

More ambitious projects have aimed at synthesizing entire genomes from scratch. In 2010, Craig Venter's group synthesized the 1-million-base-pair genome of the bacterium Mycoplasma mycoides from chemically synthesized DNA fragments, transplanted it into a cell whose original genome had been removed, and produced living, self-replicating cells whose only genetic material was the synthetic genome. The subsequent construction of a minimal genome the smallest genome sufficient to support a living cell has provided fundamental insights into the essential core of cellular life.

Metabolic engineering is the applied arm of synthetic biology redirecting cellular metabolism to produce commercially or medically valuable compounds. By introducing heterologous genes (genes from other organisms) and optimizing metabolic flux through careful pathway engineering, researchers have engineered microorganisms to produce compounds ranging from artemisinin (an anti-malarial drug originally derived from wormwood plants) to biofuels to industrial chemicals. The production of semi-synthetic artemisinin by engineered yeast, developed by Jay Keasling's group at Berkeley, has significantly increased the global supply of this drug and reduced its cost for malaria patients in developing countries.

Cell-free systems in which the transcription and translation machinery of cells is extracted and used outside of living cells offer new possibilities for rapid prototyping of synthetic biology constructs and for the on-demand production of proteins in remote or resource-limited settings. Cell-free protein synthesis has been used to produce vaccines, diagnostic reagents, and research proteins without the need for cell culture infrastructure.

12.3 Artificial Intelligence in Drug Discovery

The discovery and development of new drugs is one of the most resource-intensive endeavors in science a process that typically takes 10–15 years and costs over a billion dollars per approved drug, with an extremely high failure rate at each stage of development. Artificial intelligence, particularly deep learning, is beginning to transform this process at multiple stages.

The most dramatic early demonstration of AI's potential in structural biology came in 2020, when DeepMind's AlphaFold2 system achieved near-experimental accuracy in predicting protein three-dimensional structure from amino acid sequence alone solving a problem that had challenged structural biologists for over 50 years. The AlphaFold2 paper, published in Nature, described a deep learning architecture trained on the known database of protein structures that could predict the structure of any protein with remarkable accuracy. AlphaFold2 subsequently released predicted structures for essentially all known proteins over 200 million structures in a freely accessible database that has transformed structural biology research worldwide.

In drug discovery, AI is being applied to virtual screening the computational identification of candidate drug molecules from vast libraries of existing or hypothetical compounds. Deep learning models trained on databases of known drug-target interactions can predict which molecules are likely to bind a given target with high affinity and selectivity, dramatically reducing the number of compounds that need to be experimentally tested. AI generative models can design entirely new molecular structures optimized for specified properties potency, selectivity, metabolic stability, solubility accelerating the optimization of lead compounds.

AI is also transforming clinical development the process of testing candidate drugs in human subjects. Machine learning models applied to clinical trial data can identify patient subgroups most likely to respond to a given therapy, enabling precision medicine approaches that increase the probability of clinical success. AI analysis of electronic health records and genomic data can identify biomarkers of drug response and predict adverse effects, improving the safety and efficiency of clinical trials.

The first fully AI-designed drug candidate to enter Phase I clinical trials was DSP-1181, developed by Ex Scientia and Sumitomo Dainippon Pharma for the treatment of obsessive-compulsive disorder, in 2020. Since then, multiple AI-designed molecules have entered clinical development, and the pharmaceutical industry has made massive investments in AI-driven drug discovery platforms. The combination of CRISPR-based target validation, cryo-EM structural biology, and AI-driven drug design is creating a pipeline of unprecedented power and efficiency.

12.4 The Ethical Landscape of Biomolecular Science

The extraordinary power of modern biomolecular technologies to read and write genomes, to edit heritable human DNA, to engineer entirely new organisms, to predict protein structures and design novel drugs raises ethical questions of commensurate gravity. These are not hypothetical concerns for some distant future; they are questions that scientific and regulatory communities are grappling with right now.

Germline genome editing the modification of the genome in embryos, eggs, or sperm in ways that would be heritable by future generations is among the most controversial applications of CRISPR technology. The potential benefits are significant: germline editing could, in principle, eliminate severe inherited diseases from affected families. But the risks are equally significant: off-target edits could introduce new harmful mutations; the long-term consequences of genome edits are unknown; and the technology could potentially be misused for non-medical enhancement purposes.

The scientific and ethical consensus, as expressed by the international scientific academies and major bioethics bodies, holds that heritable human genome editing should not be attempted in clinical contexts until safety and efficacy can be demonstrated, broad societal consensus has been achieved, and appropriate regulatory oversight is in place. The case of He Jiankui the Chinese scientist who in 2018 created the first CRISPR-edited human babies, outside any regulatory framework and without community consensus was widely condemned by the scientific community as reckless and ethically indefensible, and he was sentenced to three years in prison under Chinese law.

The creation of synthetic organisms raises questions about biosafety (the risk of accidentally releasing engineered organisms into the environment) and biosecurity (the risk of deliberate misuse of synthetic biology for bioterrorism or the creation of novel pathogens). The development of oversight frameworks for synthetic biology balancing the enormous benefits of the technology against these risks is an ongoing challenge for the international scientific community and policy makers.

Data privacy is another urgent ethical issue in the omics era. Genomic data is uniquely sensitive: it reveals not only the individual's own health predispositions but those of their biological relatives. The storage, sharing, and potential misuse of genomic data by insurance companies, employers, law enforcement, and other parties poses serious privacy risks that existing legal frameworks in many countries are inadequately equipped to address.

Finally, the equitable distribution of the benefits of biomolecular technologies is a critical ethical concern. Gene therapies and CRISPR-based treatments, while transformative, currently come with price tags of millions of dollars per patient placing them completely out of reach for the vast majority of the world's population. Ensuring that the fruits of biomolecular science are accessible across economic and geographic boundaries, not only to the wealthy, is one of the great equity challenges of the coming decades.

12.5 Looking Forward: The Future of Biomolecular Science

As this book draws to a close, it is worth pausing to reflect on where biomolecular science is headed and on what its future achievements might mean for humanity.

In the near term the next decade we can anticipate the routine clinical use of CRISPR-based therapies for a growing range of genetic diseases. AlphaFold-type AI will revolutionize drug discovery, reducing the time and cost of bringing new therapeutics to patients. Single-cell omics will reveal the complete cellular architecture of human tissues and organs in health and disease. Liquid biopsies the detection of tumor-derived DNA in blood samples will enable earlier cancer diagnosis and real-time monitoring of treatment response.

In the longer term, the prospects are more speculative but potentially more transformative. Protein designs the creation of entirely new proteins with specified structures and functions is advancing rapidly, fueled by AI tools like RF diffusion and Protein MPNN. These tools can already design functional enzymes, protein nanocages, and protein-based vaccines with specified properties. The ability to design proteins at will may ultimately give us the capability to create molecular machines of arbitrary complexity molecular motors, biosensors, and therapeutic agents that nature never evolved.

Synthetic genomics the ability to design and build entire genomes from scratch raises the prospect of constructing entirely new forms of life optimized for specific applications: microorganisms that efficiently sequester carbon from the atmosphere, produce clean fuels, or manufacture complex pharmaceuticals. These possibilities come with responsibilities the careful, inclusive, and transparent governance of technologies whose implications are global.

Perhaps most fundamentally, the deepening understanding of how biomolecules interact to create life will continue to illuminate the most profound questions about what life is, how it originated, and what it means. The molecular world is not just the substrate of biology it is the foundation of mind, of memory, of perception, of emotion. Understanding it is, ultimately, a form of self-understanding.

The molecules that matter carbohydrates, lipids, proteins, nucleic acids and their diverse relatives are not merely the content of biochemistry textbooks. They are the substance of you, of every living thing that has ever existed on this planet, of life itself. To study them is to study life from the inside, with the most precise tools that science has ever developed.

This is the project to which generations of scientists have devoted their careers and their passion. It is a project that is far from finished. And the most exciting discoveries, as is always the case in science, almost certainly lie ahead.

Epilogue: The Conversation Continues

This book has taken you on a journey from the simplest atoms to the most complex molecular machines, from the structure of a glucose ring to the architecture of the CRISPR-Cas9 complex, from the folding of a single protein to the integrated metabolic networks of the living cell. Along the way, we have encountered scientists of extraordinary ingenuity Watson and Crick, Franklin, Sanger, Krebs, Mitchell, Khorana, Cech, Doudna, Charpentier, and dozens of others whose curiosity and tenacity have given us this detailed molecular map of life.

But this map, extraordinary as it is, is still incomplete. We do not fully understand how proteins fold. We do not know the complete structure and function of the human proteome. We cannot yet predict with certainty how a mutation will affect a protein's behavior in the context of a living cell. We have sequenced thousands of genomes but cannot yet interpret the function of most of the non-coding DNA that comprises the vast majority of the human genome. We do not know how the molecular events of neural activity give rise to consciousness.

These open questions are not sources of frustration but of inspiration. They are the frontier the territory where the next generation of biomolecular scientists will make their marks. If this book has conveyed the beauty of the molecular world, the excitement of discovering how life works at its most fundamental level, and the conviction that these are questions worth spending a lifetime pursuing, then it has accomplished its purpose.

The molecules that matter are waiting to be understood. The conversation between human curiosity and the molecular world continues. Welcome to the frontier.

Appendix A: Amino Acid Reference Chart

The following table lists the 20 standard amino acids used in biological protein synthesis, along with their three-letter and one-letter abbreviations, side chain class, approximate pKa values where relevant, and key structural properties.

Amino Acid	3-Letter	1-Letter	Side Chain Class	pKa (R group)	Notable Properties
Glycine	Gly	G	Non-polar, aliphatic	—	Smallest; achiral; high conformational flexibility
Alanine	Ala	A	Non-polar, aliphatic	—	Most common amino acid; hydrophobic core
Valine	Val	V	Non-polar, aliphatic	—	Branched chain; very hydrophobic; essential
Leucine	Leu	L	Non-polar, aliphatic	—	Most abundant amino acid in proteins; essential
Isoleucine	Ile	I	Non-polar, aliphatic	—	Two chiral centers; essential
Proline	Pro	P	Non-polar, cyclic	—	Secondary amine; restricts backbone flexibility; helix breaker
Phenylalanine	Phe	F	Non-polar, aromatic	—	Large aromatic ring; very hydrophobic; essential
Tryptophan	Trp	W	Non-polar, aromatic	—	Largest standard amino acid; fluorescent; essential
Methionine	Met	M	Non-polar,	—	Universal start codon amino acid; contains thioether

Amino Acid	3-Letter	1-Letter	Side Chain Class	pKa (R group)	Notable Properties
			sulfur		
Serine	Ser	S	Polar, uncharged	~13	Hydroxyl group; phosphorylation target; active site nucleophile
Threonine	Thr	T	Polar, uncharged	~13	Hydroxyl group; chiral; essential; phosphorylation target
Cysteine	Cys	C	Polar, sulfur	8.3	Thiol group; forms disulfide bonds; active site nucleophile
Tyrosine	Tyr	Y	Polar, aromatic	10.5	Phenolic OH; phosphorylation target; UV-absorbing
Asparagine	Asn	N	Polar, amide	—	Amide side chain; N-glycosylation site
Glutamine	Gln	Q	Polar, amide	—	Amide side chain; nitrogen transport in blood
Aspartate	Asp	D	Negative (acidic)	3.7	Carboxylate; key in active sites and salt bridges
Glutamate	Glu	E	Negative (acidic)	4.3	Carboxylate; neurotransmitter; enzyme active sites
Lysine	Lys	K	Positive (basic)	10.5	Epsilon-amino group; DNA binding; essential
Arginine	Arg	R	Positive (basic)	12.5	Guanidinium group; most basic; DNA binding
Histidine	His	H	Positive (basic)	6.0	Imidazole ring; pKa near physiological pH; enzyme catalysis

Appendix B: The Standard Genetic Code

The genetic code is organized by the first, second, and third bases of each codon. The table below lists all 64 codons and the amino acid (or stop signal) each encodes. Synonymous codons — those encoding the same amino acid are grouped together. Abbreviations: Stop = termination codon; Met* = start codon in addition to internal methionine.

U__ codons	**C__ codons**	**A__ codons**	**G__ codons**
UUU - Phe (F)	UCU - Ser (S)	UAU - Tyr (Y)	UGU - Cys (C)
UUC - Phe (F)	UCC - Ser (S)	UAC - Tyr (Y)	UGC - Cys (C)
UUA - Leu (L)	UCA - Ser (S)	UAA - STOP (Ochre)	UGA - STOP (Opal)
UUG - Leu (L)	UCG - Ser (S)	UAG - STOP (Amber)	UGG - Trp (W)
CUU - Leu (L)	CCU - Pro (P)	CAU - His (H)	CGU - Arg (R)
CUC - Leu (L)	CCC - Pro (P)	CAC - His (H)	CGC - Arg (R)
CUA - Leu (L)	CCA - Pro (P)	CAA - Gln (Q)	CGA - Arg (R)
CUG - Leu (L)	CCG - Pro (P)	CAG - Gln (Q)	CGG - Arg (R)
AUU - Ile (I)	ACU - Thr (T)	AAU - Asn (N)	AGU - Ser (S)
AUC - Ile (I)	ACC - Thr (T)	AAC - Asn (N)	AGC - Ser (S)
AUA - Ile (I)	ACA - Thr (T)	AAA - Lys (K)	AGA - Arg (R)
AUG - Met* (M)	ACG - Thr (T)	AAG - Lys (K)	AGG - Arg (R)
GUU - Val (V)	GCU - Ala (A)	GAU - Asp (D)	GGU - Gly (G)
GUC - Val (V)	GCC - Ala (A)	GAC - Asp (D)	GGC - Gly (G)
GUA - Val (V)	GCA - Ala (A)	GAA - Glu (E)	GGA - Gly (G)
GUG - Val (V)	GCG - Ala (A)	GAG - Glu (E)	GGG - Gly (G)

Appendix C: Glossary of Key Terms

The following glossary defines key biomolecular terms used throughout this book. Terms are listed alphabetically and cross-referenced where relevant.

Allosteric regulation: Control of enzyme activity through the binding of a regulatory molecule at a site other than the active site, inducing a conformational change that alters catalytic activity.

Alpha helix: A right-handed helical secondary structure of proteins stabilized by hydrogen bonds between backbone NH and C=O groups four residues apart; 3.6 residues per turn.

Amyloid fibril: An insoluble, highly ordered protein aggregate with a characteristic cross-beta sheet structure; associated with neurodegenerative diseases including Alzheimer's and Parkinson's.

Anomer: One of two stereoisomers of a cyclic monosaccharide that differ in configuration at the anomeric carbon (C-1); designated alpha (axial OH) or beta (equatorial OH).

Anticodon: The three-nucleotide sequence in a tRNA molecule that is complementary to and base-pairs with a specific mRNA codon during translation.

Apoptosis: Programmed cell death; a regulated process of cellular self-destruction important for development, immune function, and tumor suppression.

ATP (Adenosine triphosphate): The primary energy currency of cells; a nucleotide with three phosphate groups whose hydrolysis drives endergonic biological reactions.

Beta sheet: A secondary structure of proteins formed by hydrogen bonding between backbone groups of two or more extended polypeptide strands (beta strands) arranged side by side.

Catabolism: Metabolic processes that break down molecules and release energy, typically in the form of ATP.

Chaperone: A protein that assists in the correct folding of other proteins, preventing premature or incorrect folding and aggregation.

Chromatin: The complex of DNA and proteins (primarily histones) that constitutes chromosomes in eukaryotic cells.

Codon: A three-nucleotide sequence in mRNA that specifies a particular amino acid or a stop signal during translation.

CRISPR-Cas9: A bacterial immune system component repurposed as a precise genome editing tool; the Cas9 protein, guided by an RNA molecule, cuts double-stranded DNA at a specified target sequence.

Disulfide bond: A covalent bond formed between the sulfhydryl groups (-SH) of two cysteine residues; stabilizes extracellular protein structures.

DNA methylation: The addition of a methyl group to cytosine bases in DNA; an epigenetic modification that typically represses gene transcription.

Epigenetics: Heritable changes in gene expression that do not involve changes in the DNA nucleotide sequence; includes histone modifications and DNA methylation.

Feedback inhibition: Regulation of a metabolic pathway in which the end product inhibits an enzyme early in the pathway, controlling its own production.

Functional group: A specific arrangement of atoms in an organic molecule that confers characteristic chemical reactivity; examples include hydroxyl, carbonyl, carboxyl, amino, and phosphate groups.

Gene expression: The process by which the information encoded in a gene is used to direct the synthesis of a functional gene product (usually a protein); encompasses transcription and translation.

Genome: The complete set of genetic instructions in an organism; in eukaryotes, includes both coding and non-coding DNA sequences.

Glycolysis: The cytoplasmic pathway that converts glucose to pyruvate with net production of 2 ATP and 2 NADH per glucose molecule.

Glycoprotein: A protein with one or more covalently attached oligosaccharide chains; important in cell recognition, immune function, and protein stability.

Histone: Small, positively charged proteins around which DNA wraps to form nucleosomes, the fundamental packaging unit of eukaryotic chromatin.

Hydrophobic effect: The tendency of non-polar molecules to cluster together in aqueous solution, driven by the increase in entropy of water when non-polar surfaces are sequestered from it.

Km (Michaelis constant): The substrate concentration at which an enzyme-catalyzed reaction proceeds at half its maximum rate (Vmax); a measure of enzyme-substrate affinity.

Lipid bilayer: The fundamental structural component of cell membranes; consists of two leaflets of phospholipids arranged tail-to-tail with polar head groups facing the aqueous environment.

Metabolomics: The comprehensive analysis of small-molecule metabolites in a biological sample; provides a direct readout of the cell's current metabolic state.

Monoclonal antibody: An antibody produced by a single clone of B cells (or equivalent cell line) that recognizes a single specific antigen; widely used as research tools and therapeutic agents.

Mutation: A heritable change in the nucleotide sequence of DNA; can be a point mutation, insertion, deletion, inversion, or translocation.

Non-covalent interactions: Weak, reversible forces between molecules including hydrogen bonds, electrostatic interactions, van der Waals forces, and hydrophobic interactions; collectively responsible for molecular recognition.

Nucleosome: The basic structural unit of chromatin, consisting of approximately 147 bp of DNA wrapped 1.65 turns around a core histone octamer.

Oncogene: A gene, typically a mutated or overexpressed proto-oncogene, whose protein product promotes excessive cell proliferation and contributes to cancer development.

Oxidative phosphorylation: The process by which ATP is synthesized using the proton-motive force generated by electron transport through the inner mitochondrial membrane.

Phosphorylation: The addition of a phosphate group to a molecule, typically a protein (on Ser, Thr, or Tyr residues); a key regulatory mechanism that can activate or inactivate protein function.

Polymerase chain reaction (PCR): A technique for amplifying specific DNA sequences in vitro using repeated cycles of denaturation, primer annealing, and extension by DNA polymerase.

Proteomics: The large-scale study of the complete complement of proteins in a cell, tissue, or organism at a given time.

Ribosome: A large ribonucleoprotein complex that catalyzes the synthesis of proteins by translating mRNA sequences into polypeptide chains.

Signal transduction: The molecular process by which an extracellular signal is received by a cell surface receptor and transmitted, amplified, and converted into an intracellular response.

Splicing: The removal of non-coding intron sequences from pre-mRNA and joining of exon sequences to produce mature mRNA; carried out by the spliceosome.

Substrate: The molecule upon which an enzyme acts; it binds to the active site and is transformed into product by the enzymatic reaction.

Transcription: The process of synthesizing RNA from a DNA template, catalyzed by RNA polymerase.

Translation: The process by which the ribosome decodes the mRNA sequence and synthesizes a polypeptide chain with the specified amino acid sequence.

Tumor suppressor gene: A gene whose protein product normally restrains cell proliferation or promotes apoptosis; loss of function contributes to cancer.

Vmax: The maximum rate of an enzyme-catalyzed reaction at saturating substrate concentration; a measure of catalytic capacity.

About the Author

Abdus Salam is a scholar of biochemistry and molecular life sciences with a deep passion for making the molecular world accessible to students, researchers, and general readers alike. His academic and scientific interests span the full breadth of biomolecular science from the structural biochemistry of proteins and nucleic acids to the systems-level biology of metabolic networks and cell signaling.

Driven by the conviction that science is best communicated as the human story it is, Abdus Salam writes with equal measures of rigor and narrative engagement. His aim in this book, as in all his scientific communication, is to share the genuine wonder that the molecular world inspires in those who look closely enough and to invite a new generation of scientists to join in the extraordinary conversation between human curiosity and the machinery of life.

"The molecules that matter are waiting to be understood."

www.ingramcontent.com/pod-product-compliance
Lightning Source LLC
LaVergne TN
LVHW090409210926
848480LV00002B/506

9798233017063